T0032524

HOW TO BE HEALTHY

ANCIENT WISDOM FOR MODERN READERS
■ ■ ■ ■

For a full list of titles in the series, go to https://press.princeton.edu
/series/ancient-wisdom-for-modern-readers.

HOW TO BE HEALTHY

■ ■ ■ ■ ■

An Ancient Guide to Wellness

Galen

Selected, translated, and introduced
by Katherine D. Van Schaik

PRINCETON UNIVERSITY PRESS

PRINCETON AND OXFORD

Published by Princeton University Press
41 William Street, Princeton, New Jersey 08540
99 Banbury Road, Oxford OX2 6JX

press.princeton.edu

Library of Congress Cataloging-in-Publication Data

Names: Galen, author. | Van Schaik, Katherine D.,
editor, translator, writer of introduction.
Title: How to be healthy : an ancient guide to wellness / Galen ; selected,
translated, and introduced by Katherine D. van Schaik.
Description: Princeton : Princeton University Press, [2024] |
Series: Ancient wisdom for modern readers |
Includes bibliographical references.
Identifiers: LCCN 2023007225 (print) | LCCN 2023007226 (ebook) |
ISBN 9780691206271 (hardback) | ISBN 9780691242897 (ebook)
Subjects: LCSH: Galen—Translations into English. | Medicine, Greek
and Roman—Early works to 1800. | BISAC: PHILOSOPHY / History
& Surveys / Ancient & Classical | MEDICAL / History
Classification: LCC R126 .G48313 2024 (print) |
LCC R126 (ebook) | DDC 610.938—dc23/eng/20230703
LC record available at https://lccn.loc.gov/2023007225
LC ebook record available at https://lccn.loc.gov/2023007226

British Library Cataloging-in-Publication Data is available

Editorial: Rob Tempio and Chloe Coy
Production Editorial: Mark Bellis
Text Design: Pam Schnitter
Jacket Design: Heather Hansen
Production: Erin Suydam
Publicity: Tyler Hubbert and Carmen Jimenez
Copyeditor: Kathleen Kageff

Jacket Credit: © Archivio J. Lange / © NPL - DeA Picture
Library / Bridgeman Images

This book has been composed in Stempel Garamond LT,
Brill and Futura

Printed on acid-free paper. ∞

Printed in the United States of America

1 3 5 7 9 10 8 6 4 2

CONTENTS

The health advice contained in this book is intended for historical illumination, and while it may be timely and timeless, it is nonetheless ancient. Please consult your physician before making any drastic changes to your diet and exercise routine, or otherwise attempting to alter your humoral balance.

PREFACE

Galen is a challenging author for inclusion in the Ancient Wisdom series—which asserts (rightfully so) that classical texts provide useful, practical advice for modern readers—because so many of Galen's texts are beautifully and cohesively constructed on theories of physiology that we now know to be false. Consequently, the medical reasoning, diagnostic categories, prognoses, and therapeutic recommendations dependent on these theories are ill advised at best, and dangerous at worst. Why, therefore, should we seek wisdom in Galen's long philosophical treatises about the causes of disease, in his recommendations for preventive medicine, or in his meditations on the complex relationship between body and soul?

In fact, Galen was a careful physician and a prolix writer, offering some ancient wisdom that we today might consider modern, were it not so old. In choosing texts from the Galenic corpus for this volume, I used the following general guiding principle: I sought advice that a modern Western physician might reasonably give, or at least, with which she would not disagree (most of the time). This criterion meant that many of Galen's better-known works were excluded on this basis, as the recommendations they offer are not prescribed by today's physicians.

Drawing from nine selections from eight works, I have aggregated my chosen excerpts into five broad categories: (1) "The Mind-Body Connection," (2) "Exercising the Body," (3) "Individual Physiologies," (4) "Nourishing the Body," and (5) "Definitions of Health and Disease." Contextual information for these

categories is found at the beginning of each section. Texts in the first, second, and fourth sections ("The Mind-Body Connection," "Exercising the Body," and "Nourishing the Body") in general more straightforwardly align with my stated selection criterion. These are lively texts that, in many respects, can be practically applied to the life of a modern reader. However, it should be said that there are still some bits of text here and there, within excerpts that are broadly consistent with my theme, that would be objectionable to a modern health provider (for instance, in "On Exercise with a Small Ball," Galen's dismissal of running as a suitable form of exercise). Galen and modern physicians were and are working within—to borrow from the arguments of Thomas Kuhn—different paradigms of health and disease.[1] Their views of the human body are, in some ways, fundamentally different and completely incompatible. In this

respect, recommendation of any of Galen's texts as "an ancient guide to wellness" could be considered problematic, as such works were composed on the basis of a theoretical system that physicians no longer use.[2]

For the third and fifth sections ("Individual Physiologies" and "Definitions of Health and Disease"), my selection criterion of "advice that a modern Western physician might reasonably give, or at least, with which she would not disagree" might feel a bit inconsistent with the ideas that are presented. These selections, more philosophical in tone, make for somewhat heavier reading, and I have included them should a reader wish to see some of the theoretical foundations for the material in the other sections. I still believe that these texts are relevant for modern readers as they provide an overview of the sophistication and clarity of Galen's disease classification schemata and have,

I believe, a certain contemporary feel when considered in light of the increasing modern tendency of providers to follow diagnostic and therapeutic algorithms. Galen was constructing his diagnostic and therapeutic algorithms—if we may be allowed to use this term here—in an era without advanced laboratory and imaging techniques, but his efforts find parallels in modern endeavors to classify diseases into types and subtypes for the purpose of appropriately tailored treatment. Similarly, his focus on patients' individual constitutions and his emphasis on the necessity of the provider's acknowledgement of such particularities (highlighted in the texts in section 3) find their modern analogue in the developing field of precision medicine.

I thank Rob Tempio of Princeton University Press for his support of this approach and for his patience when the drafting of the manuscript

was delayed by the obligations of a physician practicing during a pandemic. Thanks are due, too, to Chloe Coy and other press staff, who have been helpful and encouraging throughout the process of writing and revising the manuscript. I am grateful to have been a beneficiary of Vivian Nutton's capacious knowledge of Galen and of Greco-Roman medicine; these pages reflect his thoughtful suggestions. I thank Emma Dench, Christopher Jones, Mark Schiefsky, Kathleen Coleman, Richard Thomas, and Richard Tarrant of the Harvard Department of the Classics for their many years of instruction, mentorship, and creative thinking. Christopher Parrott's patient teaching and good humor have been invaluable. My parents and brother supported an interdisciplinary course of study from the beginning; their love and encouragement propelled me through an extended and

nontraditional education. I thank Graham W. W. Van Schaik, Henry Grazioso, and James E. Crowe Jr., for reviewing the draft with the eyes of expert clinicians. James Zainaldin has helped me more than I can say; his wisdom and his comprehensive and sensitive knowledge of antiquity have improved this endeavor and many others, saving me from innumerable infelicities and errors. Finally, I thank three reviewers for the press, and copyeditor Kathleen Kageff, whose comments and corrections greatly improved the manuscript.

In the process of searching for, finding, and translating these texts, I came to believe even more strongly that excluding Galen from the Ancient Wisdom series because some of his theoretical principles do not match our own would be to deprive ourselves of a long-standing font of ancient wisdom that has served many

physicians and lay people, in many cultures, over the course of many centuries. Indeed, some of his recommendations — carefully developed from dedicated study, relentless work, and meticulous observation — remain quite sensible, even if we disagree with their theoretical foundations. Galen's close observation of the individual circumstances and physiologies of his patients, his insistence on what we today label with the terms "holistic medicine" and "wellness," and his unwavering commitment to what medical schools now call interdisciplinary medical training remain as inspiring as they ever were.

Our deepest loves nourish, enliven, and inspire us, as Galen knew well, and this book is therefore dedicated to James and to Cyrus, with great love and gratitude.

INTRODUCTION

Galen

"I am . . . extremely amazed that, although health is highly valued, men are so remiss as to neglect it: they refrain from seeking instruction in an art by which they will regain health." So the physician Galen begins his short text *On the Examinations by Which the Best Physicians Are Recognized*, written around 175 CE to teach his contemporaries how to identify a truly well-qualified physician in a world without diplomas or medical licensing boards.[3] Lamenting that educated men do not study medicine as they used to, he provides what solutions he can to this problem, outlining how someone, lacking in medical knowledge himself, could at least

identify a competent physician. The candidate should be well read in the works of his medical predecessors (including but not limited to Hippocrates, Diocles, and Praxagoras); be trained in anatomy and knowledge of the function of each organ; possess an extensive knowledge of pharmacology and dietetics; be skilled in some surgical procedures (although Galen does designate a separate set of questions to be used for interviewing surgeons); and comport himself appropriately. While it would certainly be possible *to ask* the candidate about these dimensions of his training, Galen writes, it is of course preferable *to see* him in action, successfully treating patients and predicting the course of their disease.

Galen was really describing himself and the education that he undertook, during more than a decade, to become what was surely at the time the Mediterranean world's best-trained physician.

He started practicing independently in his hometown in his late twenties and did not begin his work in Rome until his early thirties: the duration of his education is analogous to that of modern medical specialists with advanced training and secondary degrees beyond their MD certification. His knowledge, skills, experiences, oeuvre, and ego were of equally great magnitude, and we know about him and his world by dint of his own prolixity: Galen's texts constitute an estimated 10 percent of all extant Greek literature dating before 350 CE, and we know that we are still missing much of what he wrote.

The sheer volume of Galen's writing not only provided foundational principles for Western medical practice (and indeed, for much of Islamic medical practice as well) up to the nineteenth century but also gives us fascinating opportunities to peer into the daily life and world of a wealthy, well-educated Greek who

was born in modern Turkey, traveled extensively, and reached the highest echelons of the Roman Empire as a physician to the imperial family. In the nearly two millennia that have passed since Galen treated his own patients, generations of physicians, scholars, and students have gotten to know him in their own ways, focusing on many different aspects of his life and work. I include here a few of the ways that he has been described by more recent biographers and commentators, to provide a sense of the diversity of approaches used in efforts to understand this complicated, talented, and at times insufferable person. Vivian Nutton's 2020 biography is divided into chapters based on Galen's varied identities: Greek, Roman, observer, thinker, doctor, ghost (a chapter dedicated to reception history). Peter Singer's 1997 collection of English translations includes an introduction subdivided into still different identities—philosopher, "scholar and

anatomist," "systematist and inventor" — as well as a section on Galen's sophisticated views on the relationship between the body and the soul.[4] Susan Mattern's 2013 biography *The Prince of Medicine* situates Galen's development as a physician within the broader social world of the second-century Mediterranean, with a special focus on Galen's relationships with his patients. There are thousands of books and articles about Galen and his works in many languages, with still more being added annually as new manuscripts attributed to him — not only appearing in Greek but also translated into Latin, Arabic, Armenian, Hebrew, and Syriac — are uncovered in libraries, monasteries, and private collections.

Galen therefore defies simple definitions, presenting a challenge to anyone who aims to provide a brief overview of his life and work. This biographical outline therefore necessarily

overlooks details and elides nuance but hopefully provides useful background information for the texts included in this book.

Likely born in 129 CE in Pergamum (modern Bergama, Turkey), Galen was raised in a wealthy, landed family. The city of Pergamum was cosmopolitan and grand, with connections to Alexandria in Egypt, to other prominent Greek cities, and, of course, to Rome: Pergamum was an economic and cultural center in the Roman province of Asia. The city featured one of the Mediterranean's largest shrines to Asklepios (the god of healing), which may very well have influenced the young Galen's aspirations.

Galen's father, Nikon, was an architect and, by Galen's own account, a devoted father who personally taught his young son until Galen was about fourteen. The eager adolescent then began

attending lectures given by philosophers who represented a range of commitments to different schools of philosophical thought; Nikon interviewed each of them to determine their depth of knowledge and suitability as a tutor. Nikon's moderation, as Galen describes in his *Affections and Errors of the Soul*, greatly influenced Galen's own philosophical commitments and attitude toward medicine. He writes that his father's knowledge of geometry, mathematics, architecture, and astronomy led him to emphasize the importance of precision in language and to highlight the philosophical convergence around matters such as geometry and mathematics (even though there was no consensus, as such, on these topics among different philosophical and medical schools of thought). Yet Nikon also cautioned Galen not to adhere to any one philosophical sect, but rather to

scrutinize them all and to subscribe to those views most people acknowledged to be commendable and worthwhile.[5]

When Galen was sixteen, Nikon's dreams instructed him to set his talented and precocious son on a path to study not only philosophy, but also medicine. Nikon subsequently arranged for Galen to accompany at least four different physicians as they saw and treated patients in Pergamum.[6] Their backgrounds, training, and intellectual commitments were diverse, and a brief overview of the broad ideological groups to which they belonged will provide insight into Galen's training and contextualize the traditions undergirding his own way of practicing medicine.

Scholars often subdivide Greco-Roman medical practitioners of the centuries before and during Galen's lifetime into three broad groups. In this, they follow Celsus, an encyclopedist of

the first centuries BCE and CE, whose eight Latin volumes on the topic of medicine (*De Medicina*) discuss a range of topics, including the extant medical tradition, anatomy, pathophysiology, specific diseases, pharmacology, and surgical intervention. At the outset of his historical overview, Celsus writes that some physicians are committed to investigating "hidden causes" of disease, believing that proper treatment necessitates knowledge of causality.[7] These physicians were called Dogmatists or Rationalists, named for their emphasis on theories of causality. Although the practitioners in this group believed that knowledge of medical theory was crucial for successful diagnosis, treatment, and prognosis, their similarities end here: the theories to which they subscribed were remarkably diverse and generated from centuries of accumulated medical and scientific knowledge and philosophical debate. The

second broad group of physicians that Celsus describes were the Empiricists, dedicated to a tradition that focused on direct observation. When we today speak of "empirical data," we draw on this tradition of reliance on *empeiria*—a preference for allowing direct, lived experience to guide our decision making. These practitioners were impatient with what they deemed unprovable and unnecessary investigations into the hidden causes of disease and emphasized the important role of direct experience in medical training, although they did concede that, given the impossibility of encountering every medical condition in a lifetime, a physician might have recourse to the writings of reliable predecessors in uncertain or newly encountered cases. Galen's teachers in Pergamum fell into—and straddled the line between—these two broad groups of physicians (the Rationalists/Dogmatists and the

Empiricists). The third group of physicians that Celsus describes, the Methodists, were also averse to theorizing about etiology. They sorted diseases into three broad categories (excessive looseness, excessive constriction, and a mixed state). This medical sect, in particular, attracted Galen's ire, and its practitioners were often the targets of vitriolic abuse in his texts and public demonstrations.

The young Galen's four and possibly five physician teachers in Pergamum represented a wide range of medical epistemologies. Definitely one teacher (Aeschrion) and possibly a second (Epicurus) were Empiricists, whose perspectives must have deeply influenced Galen's own practice. In his later writings, Galen describes his admiration for the Empiricists' careful attention to detail, and he praises their focus on direct experience and repeated observation, including their extensive descriptions of the

pulse. Yet, he objected to the Empiricist stance against deductive and causal reasoning. Galen's own extensive corpus is evidence of his commitment to a theoretical framework that did involve these kinds of reasoning, even as his views on medical training shared the Empiricist emphasis on observation and *empeiria*.

Galen's additional physician teachers in Pergamum would have been classified as Dogmatists/Rationalists, although Empiricist practices likely influenced them, too. One of them, a Pneumatist, would have seen imbalances in *pneuma* (breath that was physiologically modified by the heart and brain) as a cause of disease. Satyrus, himself a student of the famous physician Quintus, was an especially important teacher for Galen and does not seem to have aligned himself with any particular medical sect, although he appears to have taken an Empiricist approach to many dimensions of medical education and

practice. Bringing the teenage Galen along to treat patients, Satyrus instructed him in anatomy and pharmacology, inspiring his eager pupil to seek out other students of Quintus on the travels he would begin to undertake in his twenties, after his father's death.

The practical dimension of Galen's medical education was augmented by his indefatigable commitment to reading as much of the enormous written medical tradition as he could. Like the dedicated premedical students in the modern American university, Galen matter-of-factly (and perhaps hubristically) states that he outstudied his fellow pupils, devoting days and nights to the development of his medical acumen. He quotes the texts of his medical predecessors throughout his work, often to point out their flaws. Above all, he draws on the Hippocratic Corpus, celebrating Hippocrates as the ideal and foundational physician. Galen's

own theories of physiology and medical practice drew heavily on the Hippocratic Corpus, even as he presented his own modifications of it. Indeed, as the teenage Galen was reading and studying the works of his predecessors, he was also composing his own texts. He wrote three books during his early period of medical study in Pergamum: a description of the anatomy of the uterus (which survives in Greek), a treatise on eye diseases (surviving in fragments in Arabic), and a description of a debate between Empiricist and Hippocratic physicians (surviving in Arabic).

After Nikon died, when Galen was eighteen or nineteen, Galen set out on his decade-long educational journey around the Mediterranean before eventually returning to Pergamum in 157 CE. A highlight of Galen's travels involved a prolonged stay in Alexandria, which had for centuries been recognized as a center

of medical learning. It was here, from the late 300s BCE to the mid 200s BCE, that physician-scientists Herophilus and Erasistratus had undertaken groundbreaking dissections of human cadavers, radically changing existing assumptions about the human body and inspiring increased emphasis on the value of anatomy in medical training.[8] Although systematic dissections on human cadavers would not occur again until the late Renaissance, the new knowledge generated through Herophilus's and Erasistratus's activities made Galen, among others, a strong proponent of the value of anatomy in medical training and continuing education. Galen would, throughout his life and often in public, dissect pigs, primates, sheep, and goats to further refine his anatomical knowledge and to demonstrate his medical and technical skills. He never dissected humans, but, in both his training and his medical practice, he explicitly took the opportunity

to note the internal human anatomy he encountered when treating traumatic injuries and conducting surgeries.

Back in Pergamum in 157 CE, Galen served as the physician for the professional gladiators who fought in ceremonial games honoring the Roman imperial cult, a role that might find its rough modern equivalent in being the team physician or head orthopedist for a top-notch basketball or football team. The analogy is only an approximate one, however: he secured this role in a grisly public display of his prowess in front of the chief priest responsible for selecting the gladiators' physician. Galen cut open the abdomen of a monkey and challenged his competitors for the position to replace its entrails and close the wound. When these other candidates did nothing (as Galen tells us), he took up his own challenge, thereby securing the prestigious position he sought. He would not have

disappointed the chief priest who selected him for the role: he tells us that only two gladiators died during his first year on the job. He also notes that none of them died during the remaining four years of his tenure. His predecessor, Galen points out, failed to save sixteen of these well-trained and expensive athletes. In addition to treating serious traumatic injuries, he was responsible for overseeing more mundane aspects of their health, such as their diet.

Given Galen's ambitions and agonistic spirit, it is not surprising that he made his way to Rome in 162 CE, where his talents were noticed by social elites and prominent government officials when he successfully treated one of their mutual friends shortly after his arrival. Galen was invited to give public demonstrations of his prowess, including dissections of animals, and to treat wealthy and powerful Romans and their families. A parallel might be drawn to modern

concierge medicine. Galen was, by his own account, at least, an in-demand physician and a supremely talented and successful surgeon, in particular.

This first stay in Rome was relatively short, as Galen departed in 166 CE. He writes that he was driven out by jealous rivals, but it is also likely that the outbreak of plague in Asia Minor may have prompted him to want to return home to help. He sailed from Rome back to Pergamum, picking up plants and minerals for therapeutic use en route. But the thirty-nine-year-old Galen was called back to Italy in 168 CE by none other than the Roman emperor himself, who required his services while on a military campaign against the Germanic tribes who were making their way to northern Italy.

Galen departed Pergamum, and after arriving in Aquileia, the staging ground for the Roman army near the modern border of Italy and

Slovenia, found himself face to face with the plague (possibly smallpox, or another related virus). If Galen contracted the disease, he does not mention it in the sources that we have. Susan Mattern offers the intriguing suggestion that Galen's experiences dissecting and vivisecting animals may have inoculated him against the disease through exposure to a related poxvirus, much in the way that English physician Edward Jenner, of the late eighteenth and early nineteenth centuries, used effluvia of cowpox pustules to vaccinate (*vacca* is, of course, Latin for "cow") his patients against smallpox.[9]

Back in Rome in 169 CE and treating wealthy and well-connected patients as he had done previously, Galen was asked by the emperor Marcus Aurelius to set out with the army again. A dream from Asklepios advised against this, Galen told the pious Marcus Aurelius, who permitted Galen to remain in Rome to oversee the

production of the drug theriac and to serve as a court physician to his son Commodus.[10] This period was an immensely productive one for Galen, who wrote many of his most comprehensive works during this time. When Marcus Aurelius died in 180, however, a period of disruption ensued. Many of Galen's friends lost their lives and property in the subsequent civil strife. Perhaps the greatest tragedy of Galen's own life came in 192 CE, when an enormous fire destroyed the Temple of Peace and its environs, including much of the Palatine Hill. This wealthy area of Rome contained well-appointed homes, extensive library collections, and, sadly for Galen, storehouses where he kept his irreplaceable manuscripts, plants, and minerals from his decades of travel, and even bespoke surgical instruments made from especially high-quality metal. An excerpt of the text Galen composed to tell an old friend how he coped

with such a loss (*Avoiding Distress*) is included in this volume.

Less is known about the later decades of Galen's life. It seems that after the assassination of Commodus in 192 CE, Galen continued to practice, to teach, and to write, with a focus on recomposing texts lost in the fire or trying to obtain copies of versions he had previously shared with friends. In these last years of his life, he may have stayed in Rome, or he could have returned to Pergamum. The date of his death is not known with certainty but estimated by later Arabic sources to be around 216 CE, when he was approximately eighty-seven years old.

Works and Theories of Physiology

Galen wrote seemingly unceasingly. His extant texts are characterized by their commitment to the creation and consolidation of a unified presentation of health and disease that

encompasses his own interpretations of the theoretical commitments of his predecessors, the anatomical and pathophysiological details they recorded, and his own personal experience. They are also undeniably self-promotional and deeply vitriolic against those with whom he disagrees, or those whom he perceives to question his authority and skill. Yet, we cannot help but marvel at his capacious intellect, limitless curiosity, and unquestionable work ethic. He wrote about food, anatomy and dissection, physiology, philosophy, surgeries (on all parts of the body), bodily functions (including the pulse, breathing, and mechanisms of smell and movement), pharmacology, bandaging techniques, exercise, fertility and embryology, the history of medicine up to his own day, techniques of diagnosis and prognosis, mental health and disease, and assessment of bodily fluids, besides commentaries on the works of earlier writers

(including Hippocrates and Plato), philosophical texts, and reflections on his own knowledge, training, and experiences. The overarching unity of his theories of health and disease and the nuance with which he could fit his experiences and observations into his intellectual framework mean that any brief summary of his theories is an oversimplification—and probably one to which he would have strenuously objected. But, I will attempt such a summary here, so that the included texts might be understood within the context of Galen's broader oeuvre.

Anatomical dissections had convinced Galen that three separate systems, guided by the brain, the heart, and the liver, were responsible for the functioning of the human body. The liver processed (a frequent translation of the Greek is "concocted," meaning "to cook together") ingested food, turning it into blood, which traveled through the veins to nourish all the other

parts of the body. The heart served as a kind of waystation, taking this nutritious venous blood into its right side and, via the interventricular septum, combining it with air (*pneuma*) that entered the left side of the heart through the pulmonary vein, along with a small amount of blood. This conclusion about the functioning of the heart, although obviously wrong to us today, took into account earlier observations of the Alexandrian anatomists.[11] The left side of the heart concocted this mixture of blood and pneuma, yielding a refined red blood that lent its "vital spirit" to the rest of the body via the arteries. The vessels in the brain refined this special blood still further, mixing it with air inhaled through the nostrils to yield "psychic pneuma" (the pneuma connected with the *psychē*, or soul), which nourished the brain and nerves that Galen and many of his predecessors recognized to be the key anatomical

parts responsible for movement, sensation, and consciousness.

In constructing his physiology, Galen built on Hippocratic, Aristotelian, and other scientific and medical theories involving balance of the elements (air, fire, water, earth), seasons (spring, summer, autumn, winter), and humors (blood, yellow bile, phlegm, black bile).[12] Each patient had his or her own ideal, individual balance of these humors; this may or may not have been the same as a general, ideal balance of all four. Disease states represented deviations from this individual personal balance, and patients would have proclivities to certain afflictions based on that particular balance. This framework provided the theoretical foundation for therapies (such as modifications of diet and exercise, changes of location, and use of pharmacological compounds or more invasive therapies such as bleeding) to bring an individual's

particular balance back to its natural state when an external influence (including psychological stress) disrupted it. Although varying widely in their subject matter, Galen's many texts assume this basic framework in their discussion and recommendations.

A Brief Comment on Citations, Textual Editions, and Translations

Galen's manuscript tradition—that is, the actual physical manuscripts that scribes copied and re-copied, which we now use as the sources of the texts attributed to Galen—is very complicated. Many of these precious texts exist only in a single manuscript, which itself may be in poor condition, copied by a scribe who clearly intro-duced errors as he wrote out the text we have, using another copy that we no longer have. In other cases, multiple manuscripts of a text may exist, but they may not all include the same parts

of the text, or they may have discrepancies or be written in different languages (none of which are Greek)—or all the above. These challenges mean that the Greek texts we see neatly printed in this book are the product of much effort and frequent disagreements among talented papyrologists, philologists, and historians.

The most comprehensive collection of Galen's work was published between 1821 and 1833 by the German pathologist and physiologist Carl Gottlob Kühn. Yet his compilation of Galen's work is not without errors, and for many texts, his edition has been superseded because new manuscripts of Galen's work have since been found that have improved our understanding of previous texts. However, the enduring existence of Kühn's collection, its relative accessibility, and its status as a frame of reference for so many textual critics and scholars mean that citations to Galen's texts invariably

will include the associated reference to Kühn, along with other citations to more up-to-date and likely more accurate versions of the text. In each case in this book, if there is a Kühn text, I have provided my chosen primary source for the Greek text, the corresponding citation in the Kühn text, and any changes that I have made to the Greek on the basis of consultations of other editions and translations. Numbers within the text correspond to the volume and page number of the Kühn edition of that text; for example, a reference to volume 6, page 304, line 3 of Kühn's text will be written "6.304.3K" in parentheses in both the Greek text and the English translation. At the start of the text, I have provided the volume, page, and line number of the Kühn text. Subsequent references in the text note the start of each page of Kühn. In some cases, if I have used a text besides that of Kühn, I have also provided the numbering system for

that edition, while using Kühn as the primary numerical reference. I have done this for ease of reading and reference, as the use of multiple numbering systems simultaneously can be confusing, especially for those unaccustomed to the Galenic textual tradition. There are more comprehensive notes on each selection in the back-matter section "Source Texts."

As I discuss further in my cautionary note below, translation of any text is challenging, especially those that draw on a technical vocabulary that is still used today, albeit in different forms and with different meanings. Galen prided himself on being a philosopher, steeped in the traditions of Plato, Aristotle, the Stoics, and many others. His Greek reflects this philosophical education, and he makes fine distinctions among categories, carefully explaining definitions and boundaries. His tone, diction, and grammatical structures might be described as

"professorial," and I have attempted to capture these aspects of his writing in English. At the same time, I have tried to strike a balance between the literal rendering that conveys Galen's technical but stylized prose, and a sometimes freer translation that privileges ease of reading and understanding for a modern, general audience. References to other English translations of each text are provided so that readers might see other ways of interpreting Galen's Greek, if they so desire. In preparing my own translations, I have consulted, in particular, translations by Ian Johnston and Peter Singer. Full references to these works are found in the section "Further Reading" at the end of this volume.

Regarding transliterations of Greek to English in notes and comments, I have followed standard conventions for all words except proper names, in which case I have used (for the most

part) Latinized versions, as they are typically more familiar to general audiences.

A Final Cautionary Note: Health, Disease, and Ancient and Modern Comparisons

There is, I think, a particular joy that comes from recognizing emotions and moments in our own modern lives in the words and remains of people who lived so long ago. Such experiences are affirming for one's humanity and motivate study of the past in a way that is deeply personal. Matters of sickness and health, especially, can foster such cross-chronological connections as we ponder the shared experience of living in an aging human body that can be both frail and resilient.

However, these obvious connections that we have with people in the past can also lead us to engage reflexively in retrospective diagnosis, the

process by which we seek to impose modern diagnostic terms and categories on historical records of disease. Such activities can be problematic for several reasons, a few of which I will list here. First, diagnosis involves the examination of a patient and discussion of the patient's symptoms, which are obviously not possible in the case of someone who lived two thousand years ago. Second, notions of normal and abnormal are variable, even within the same medical tradition, during the same time period: presented with such diagnostic gray areas in our own context, we should be sensitive to their presence in other contexts, as well. Third, modern medical terminology in the Western tradition uses Greek and Latin terms. This is a boon to the medical student who has studied Greek and Latin but can be deceptive for the incautious reader of ancient Greco-Roman medical texts. Although modern physicians use diagnostic

labels from Greek words (e.g., *pneumonia*, *ascites*, *carcinoma*), such labels, when encountered in ancient texts, may or may not designate the pathological processes a modern Western physician associates with these terms. The Greco-Roman medical tradition is long, and such terms were used differently by different authors, writing in variable geographic locations and subscribing to different schools of thought and practice, over centuries. Some authors even used terms inconsistently within their own texts, or their use of such terms evolved with time. (Detailed overviews of Galen's terminology may be found in Singer's and Johnston's translations.) Such variation advises caution in how we interpret these terms in ancient medical texts.

Fourth, the burdens of disease (the broad range of conditions, injuries, and disabilities experienced by a given population within a certain

time period) in Galen's world and in our world are very different. Galen formed his recommendations on the basis of observations made in an environment with higher rates of malnutrition, maternal and fetal mortality, child mortality, and irreparable traumatic injury compared to rates of those conditions in developed nations today. In Galen's Mediterranean world, even small, localized infections or a simple diarrheal illness could be fatal. There were no vaccines, antibiotics, or anesthesia (aside from alcohol and opium). Although people did, like Galen, live to quite advanced ages, most did not, and average life expectancy at birth was not above forty years. Bioarchaeological study of human remains does provide evidence for the occurrence of diseases that we consider chronic or related to long life, like atherosclerosis and cancer, but it can be next to impossible to identify these pathologies, as we understand them,

through written records alone. Attention to the vast differences in the disease burdens of the ancient world and of the modern developed world both provides a useful lens through which to understand Galen's own perspective and reminds us not to form hasty diagnostic conclusions about the people and pathologies we encounter in his texts.

These caveats are not presented in order to say that the identification of pathological processes in historical records of disease is impossible; impressive advances in technology, merged with detailed linguistic and historical analysis, have yielded striking insights into the health and disease of past populations and have confirmed the presence—even down to the genetic sequence—of many pathogens. But such processes are undertaken by interdisciplinary teams of experts who, ideally, bring to the discussion recognition of the respective limitations of each

of their own analytical techniques. Many pursuing these interdisciplinary questions of health and disease in past populations prefer the phrase "retrospective differential diagnosis," which qualifies conclusions by providing a range of plausible diagnoses, instead of pointing to a single, narrowly defined possibility.

We know more than we ever have about health and disease in the past, but this does not obviate an approach to ancient medical texts that recognizes that they describe a world different from our own. In fact, such knowledge leads us to the conclusion that, in spite of these differences, we can still connect with and be inspired by the achievements that such ancient texts represent and the human compassion they evoke.

TEXTS AND TRANSLATIONS

1

The Mind-Body Connection

Galen's views on the *psychē* (itself a word with broad meanings in Greek, some of which correspond to the concepts of "mind," "soul," and perhaps "life force" in English) are a complex, unique amalgamation of his own anatomical investigations and clinical experiences, the recorded observations and theories of his predecessors, and philosophical (especially Platonic, but also Aristotelian) thought. An excellent overview of this complicated topic and its relationship with the broader intellectual milieu in which Galen learned and wrote may be found in Singer's 2013 volume *Galen: Psychological Writings*. In brief, as Singer argues, Galen described his views on the physiological, mechanistic

interrelationship of the body and the soul primarily in a text he wrote in an earlier phase of his career, *The Doctrines of Hippocrates and Plato*. Some of these ideas are further explored in a later work, *The Capacities of the Soul Depend on the Mixtures of the Body*. The selections included here come not from these more technical texts, but instead from treatises he focused on near the end of his life. They highlight Galen's sensitivity to patients' mental needs and demonstrate how he applies philosophical concepts in a practical way to improve patients' (and his own) mental health. These texts also show his awareness of the connection between mental and physical health, a concept that has been the subject of increased investigation in modern medical research. His recommendations regarding emotional regulation, contextualization of loss, and the importance of continued efforts toward self-improvement are commonly

encountered in psychological and therapeutic approaches today.

Avoiding Distress

This recently discovered (2005) text intimately describes Galen's method for coping with emotionally challenging circumstances, including references to the great personal losses he sustained in the fire of 192 CE. Although "Avoiding Distress" has been known to scholars for less than twenty years, there have been multiple editions offering their own subtle changes to the original Greek text, a consequence of a poor-quality manuscript whose owners have restricted scholars' access to it. I have primarily followed the text of the Budé edition, with some changes (indicated with endnotes) that reflect Garofalo's emendations and Nutton's English translation. The addressee is probably a longtime friend of Galen's from his hometown,

(38) Ἴσως ἂν οὖν φήσεις ἐπιτάττεσθαί σου τὴν ἐπι-
θυμίαν καὶ βούλεσθαι μᾶλλον γνῶναι πῶς ἀπολέσας
τοσαύτην ποικιλίαν κτημάτων ὧν ἕκαστον αὐτὸ καθ᾽
ἑαυτὸ μόνον λυπηρότατον ἂν ἐγένετο τοῖς ἄλλοις ἀνθρώποις, οὐκ ἠνιάθην ὡς ἕτεροί τινες, ἀλλὰ πάνυ
<ῥᾳδίως> ἤνεγκα τὸ συμβάν. **(39)** Ἐγὼ δέ σοι διττὴν
ἀπόκρισιν πρὸς τοῦτο ποιήσομαι, τὴν μὲν ἑτέραν
ὑπὲρ ἧς ἀναμνησθῆναί σε χρὴ πολλάκις ἀκηκοότα δι-
ερχομένου <ἐμοῦ> τοιούτους λόγους ὧν καὶ νῦν ἄρξο-
μαι τῆς ἀναμνήσεως·

*Pergamum, and the letter was probably writ-
ten in early to mid-193 CE. Epicurean, Stoic,
Aristotelian, and Platonic elements can be
found in the advice Galen offers, which is all
the more moving because, as he argues, it has
worked for him.*

A DOCTOR'S ADVICE FOR COPING WITH LOSS, FROM PERSONAL EXPERIENCE

(38) Maybe you will say that your desire has
been spurred onward and that you want to
know more about how I, when I lost so many
possessions—the loss of each of which on its
own would have been incredibly upsetting to
other men—was not distressed by it as other
men would be, but instead tolerated the accident
very easily. (39) I will give you two reasons for
this, one of which you must remember, since
often you heard me discussing anecdotes of the
sort with which I now begin my recollection.

φιλότιμος Ἀρίστιππος, οὐκ ἀρκούμενος διαίτῃ
εὐτελεῖ ἀλλὰ καὶ πολυτελείαις ὄψων [ἂν] ἑκάστης
ἡμέρας διδοὺς ἀργύριον ἑκάστοτε δαψιλὲς τοῖς θερ-
μοτέροις τῶν κατ᾽ αὐτὸν ἑταίρων—ὅμως καί τι πολλῶν δεόμενος ὁ ἀνὴρ ἐκεῖνος—, (40) ἀνιών ποτε ἐκ
Πειραιῶς—εἰώθει ἀεὶ βαδίζειν οὐ μόνον τὰς οὕτω
βραχείας ὁδούς, ἀλλὰ καὶ τὰς μακράς—, ἐπειδὴ
ἐθεάσατο τὸν οἰκέτην μὴ δυνάμενον ἕπεσθαι τῷ
φορτίῳ—φασκώλιον δὲ ἦν τοῦτο χρυσίων μεστόν—,
ἐκέλευσεν ἀποχέαι τοσοῦτον ὡς τὸ λοιπὸν εὔφορον
αὐτῷ γενέσθαι. (41) Κατὰ τὴν αὐτὴν οὖν γνώμην
ἔπραξε καὶ τόδε· τέσσαρας ἔχων ἀγροὺς ἐπὶ τῆς πα-
τρίδος, ἕνα κατά τινα περίστασιν τῶν πραγμάτων ἐξ
αὐτῶν ἀπήλασεν ὡς λοιπὸν ἔχειν τρεῖς. (42) Ἀπαν-
τήσας οὖν τις τῶν πολιτῶν ἕτοιμος* ἦν ἐπὶ τῇ ζημίᾳ
συλλυπεῖσθαι· γελάσας οὖν ὁ Ἀρίστιππος ἔφη· "τί

---

* I here use the reading ἕτοιμος of Garofalo and Lami, *Galeno: L'anima e il dolore*, and of Nutton CMG V 8,1, *Galeni De Praecognitione*, instead of the reading οἷος of Boudon-Millot, Jouanna, and Pietrobelli, *Galien*, vol. 4, *Ne pas se chagriner*.

The profligate Aristippus, not content with a thrifty lifestyle, frequently gave large sums of money to host extravagant daily feasts for the more zealous among his pupils—but there were many things that even he did not have. **(40)** One day, as he was coming back from the Piraeus (it was his custom always to walk, not only for short trips like this one, but also for longer ones), when he saw that his servant was unable to hold on to his burden (his little bag was full of gold), he ordered the servant to take out as much of the gold as needed to make the remaining burden easy to carry. **(41)** In the same frame of mind, he also did this: although he had four fields in his hometown, he lost one of them because of some difficulties in his affairs, with the result that he had three left. **(42)** One of his fellow citizens, coming to meet him, was eager to show his sympathy for the loss. Aristippus

μᾶλλον ἐμοὶ <σὺ> συλλυπήσῃ τρεῖς ἀγροὺς ἔχοντι
τοιούτους οἷον <ἕνα> μόνον αὐτὸς ἔχεις ἢ ἐγώ σοι
συλλυπήσομαι;"

πάνυ καλῶς ἐνδεικνύμενος ὃ πολλάκις ἤκουσας
παρ᾽ ἐμοῦ λεγόμενον ὡς οὐ χρὴ πρός τι τῶν ἀπολλυ-
μένων ἐμβλέπειν καὶ λογίζεσθαι πῶς οἱ τρεῖς ἀγροὺς
δεξάμενοι τοῦ πατρὸς οὐκ ἀνέξονται βλέπειν ἑτέρους
ἔχοντας τριάκοντα· (43) καὶ γὰρ ἐὰν τριάκοντα
ἔχωσιν, ἑτέρους ὄψονται πεντήκοντα ἔχοντας· ἐὰν
<κατὰ> ταὐτὰ πάλιν αὐτοὶ κτήσωνται τοσούτους,
ἔχοντας ὄψονταί τινας ἄλλους ἑβδομήκοντα, κἂν
ἐκείνους ἔχωσιν, ἄλλους θεάσονται πλείους τῶν ἑκα-
τὸν ἔχοντας, ὥστε κατὰ βραχὺ προϊόντες ἁπάντων
ἐπιθυμήσουσιν, καὶ κατὰ τοῦτο ἀεὶ πένητες ἔσονται,
μὴ πληρουμένης αὐτῶν τῆς ἐπιθυμίας.

laughed and said, "Why should you show me sympathy, when I have three of these kinds of fields, while you only have one? Or should I be showing you sympathy?"

He very finely demonstrates what you have heard me say very often: you should not fixate on what was lost, and you should consider how men who have received three fields from their father cannot stand to look at other people who have thirty fields. **(43)** For in fact if they have thirty, they will focus on other people who have fifty. Again, if in the same way they will obtain as many, then they will focus on others who have seventy fields, and even if they have these, they will see others who have more than a hundred, with the result that, proceeding little by little like this, they will covet everything. In this way, they will always be poor because their longing is insatiable.

(44) Ἐὰν δέ τις μὴ πόσους ἀγροὺς ἄλλος ἔχει διὰ τέλους σκοπῇ, ἀλλ' ἤ<δη> τοὺς ἰδίοις ἀναλώμασιν ἐξαρκοῦντας αὐτῷ, τὴν τῶν περιττωμάτων ἀπώλειαν ἀκηδῶς οἴσει. (45) Ἐὰν μὲν γάρ τις ἕνα μόνον ἔχων ἀγρὸν ἀπολέσῃ τοῦτον, ἄπορο<ς> ἔσται παντάπασιν, ὥστε εἰκότως ἀνιαθήσεται, ἕνα δὲ ἀπολέσας <τις> ἐκ τῶν τεσσάρων, ἐν ἴσῳ καταστήσεται τοῖς τρεῖς ἔχουσιν ἐξ ἀρχῆς, ὥστε τούτῳ μὲν μέγα οὐδὲν μὴ λυπεῖσθαι τρεῖς ἀγροὺς ὑπολοίπους ἔχοντι, μέγα δὲ τὸ τὸν μηδὲ ἕνα κεκτημένον ἀγρὸν ἀλύπως φέρειν πενίαν ὡς ὁ Κράτης ἔφερε, καὶ διὰ τοῦτο μᾶλλον εἴ <τις> μηδὲ οἰκίαν ἔχει[ν] καθάπερ ὁ Διογένης. (46) Οὐκοῦν ἐμοὶ τί πρᾶγμα μέγα μηδ' ὅλως ἀνιαθέντι διὰ χρημάτων ἀπώλειαν; Ἦν γὰρ ἀεὶ τὰ λειπόμενα πολὺ πλέω τῶν ἱκανῶν.

(44) But, if someone is not forever keeping an eye on how many fields someone else has, but instead looks to what suffices for his own expenses, he will bear the loss of the excess with indifference. **(45)** On the other hand, if someone with a single field loses it, then he will be totally without means and will reasonably be distressed. But someone who lost one of his four fields is in the same position as those who had three from the beginning, so it is no great thing for the man who still has three fields not to be upset. But it is a great thing for the man who never owned a field to endure his poverty without distress, as Crates endured it, and for that reason an even greater thing if he never had even a house, like Diogenes.[13] **(46)** So really, it was no great affair for me to be wholly unperturbed at the loss of my property, for what remains is much more than enough.

Affections and Errors of the Soul

This text, likely written later in Galen's life, is part of the tradition of practical ethics, the idea that philosophical concepts could positively and productively affect one's mental state and behavior. The philosophical origins of such therapy for the soul may be found in multiple schools of thought, including Stoicism, Epicureanism, Platonism, and Aristotelianism (as is the case for much of Galen's work). Although there are many affections about which one could be concerned—among them rage, anger,

fear, distress, envy, and excessive desire—in this text, Galen focuses especially on anger and distress. The excerpt appears in the beginning of the treatise, when he is making a distinction between affections, which he argues have a more irrational component, and errors, which are more aligned with rational capacities (although these distinctions are not perfect or absolute). Galen addresses the work to someone who must have been one of his oldest friends, who shared his political views and maintained a relationship with him despite the distance that likely separated them.

(**4.2D = 5.2.14K**) ἐγὼ δ' αὐτὸ τοῦτο πρῶτον, ὡς οἶσθα, διώρισα, τὸ μὲν ἁμάρτημα κατὰ ψευδῆ (**4.4D = 5.3K**) δόξαν εἰπὼν γίγνεσθαι, τὸ δὲ πάθος κατά τιν' ἄλογον ἐν ἡμῖν δύναμιν ἀπειθοῦσαν τῷ λόγῳ· κοινῇ δ' ἀμφότερα κατὰ <τὸ> γενικώτερον σημαινόμενον ἁμαρτήματα κεκλῆσθαι. λέγομεν οὖν ἁμαρτάνειν καὶ τὸν ἀκολασταίνοντα καὶ τὸν θυμῷ τι πράττοντα καὶ τὸν διαβολῇ πιστεύοντα.

γέγραπται μὲν οὖν καὶ Χρυσίππῳ καὶ ἄλλοις πολλοῖς τῶν φιλοσόφων θεραπευτικὰ γράμματα τῶν τῆς ψυχῆς παθῶν, εἴρηται δὲ καὶ πρὸς Ἀριστοτέλους <περὶ τούτων> καὶ τῶν ἑταίρων αὐτοῦ καὶ πρὸ τούτων ὑπὸ Πλάτωνος· καὶ ἦν μὲν βέλτιον ἐξ ἐκείνων μανθάνειν αὐτά, ὥσπερ κἀγώ. τὰ δ' οὖν κεφάλαια διὰ τοῦ πρώτου λόγου τοῦδε διὰ συντόμου, ἐπειδὴ κελεύεις, διήξω σοι πάντα, καθ' ἣν ἤδη τάξιν

(4.2D = 5.2.14K) From the very first, I made this distinction, that an error occurs in accordance with false **(4.4D = 5.3K)** belief,[14] and that affection[15] occurs according to some irrational faculty in us that does not comply with reason; colloquially, both in a more general sense are called errors. So, we say that someone has erred when he behaves dissolutely, or does something from anger, or believes a false accusation.

Chrysippus and many other philosophers have written therapeutic texts for affections of the soul, and Aristotle and his followers, and Plato before them, also discussed these things. It would be better to learn these things from them, as I did. So, in this first section, I will set out for you the main points in an abridged form, since you are requesting that I do so, according

ἤκουσας, ὅτ' ἐπύθου περὶ τοῦ γεγραμμένου τῷ Ἀντωνίῳ βιβλίου.

Ὅτι μὲν εἰκός ἐστιν ἁμαρτάνειν, εἰ καὶ μὴ δοκοίημεν αὐτοὶ σφάλλεσθαί τι, πάρεστιν ἐκ τῶνδε λογίσασθαι· πάντας ἀνθρώπους ὁρῶμεν ἑαυτοὺς ὑπολαμβάνοντας ἤτοι γε ἀναμαρτήτους εἶναι παντάπασιν ἢ ὀλίγα καὶ σμικρὰ καὶ διὰ πολλοῦ σφάλλεσθαι, καὶ τοῦτο (4.20D = 5.4K) μάλιστα πεπονθότας, οὓς ἄλλοι πλεῖστα νομίζουσιν ἁμαρτάνειν. ἐγὼ γοῦν, εἰ καί τινος ἑτέρου, καὶ τοῦδε παμπόλλην ἔσχηκα πεῖραν· ὅσοι μὲν τῶν ἀνθρώπων [ἐπ'] ἄλλοις ἐπέθεντο τὴν περὶ αὐτῶν ἀπόφα<ν>σιν, ὁποῖοί τινές εἰσιν, ὀλίγα τούτους ἐθεασάμην ἁμαρτάνοντας, ὅσοι δ' ἑαυτοὺς ὑπειλήφασιν ἀρίστους εἶναι χωρὶς τοῦ τὴν κρίσιν ἑτέροις ἐπιτρέψαι, μέγιστα καὶ πλεῖστα τούτους ἑώρακα σφαλλομένους.

ὥσθ' ὅπερ ᾤμην, ὅτε μειράκιον ἦν, ἐπαινεῖσθαι μάτην τοῦτο δ' ἦν τὸ Πύθιον γνῶναι κελεῦον ἑαυτόν· οὐ γὰρ εἶναι μέγα τὸ πρόσταγμα, τοῦθ' εὗρον ὕστερον

to the arrangement you heard before, when you asked about Antonius's book.

That we are probably making mistakes even if we ourselves believe that we are not slipping up can be readily gathered from the following: we see that all assume that they are without error entirely, or that they make a few small errors rarely, and that it is **(4.20D = 5.4K)** above all those who think this way whom others believe err the most. I have also learned the following through my experience as much as anything else: men who enjoin others to point out their errors are the sort of people whom I have rarely witnessed making mistakes, but those who assume that they are the best without entrusting judgement to others I have seen slipping up most and most often.

As a young man, I used to think that the Pythian oracle's command "Know thyself" was overrated, since I did not think it was any

δικαίως ἐπαινούμενον. ἀκριβῶς μὲν γὰρ ὁ σοφώτα-
τος μόνος ἂν ἑαυτὸν γνοίη, τῶν δ' ἄλλων ἁπάντων
ἀκριβῶς μὲν οὐδείς, ἧττον δὲ καὶ μᾶλλον ἕτερος ἑτέρου. καθάπερ γὰρ ἐν ὅλῳ τῷ βίῳ καὶ κατὰ πάσας
τὰς τέχνας τὰς μὲν μεγάλας ὑπεροχάς τε καὶ δια-
φορὰς τῶν πραγμάτων ἅπαντος ἀνδρός ἐστι γνῶναι,
τὰς δὲ μικρὰς τῶν φρονίμων τε καὶ τεχνιτῶν, οὕτω
κἀπὶ τῶν ἁμαρτημάτων ἔχει (5.9D = 5.5K) καὶ
παθῶν. ὅστις μὲν ἐπὶ μικροῖς ὀργιζόμενος σφοδρῶς
δάκνει τε καὶ λακτίζει τοὺς οἰκέτας, οὗτος μέν σοι
δῆλός ἐστιν ἐν πάθει καθεστηκώς, ὁμοίως δὲ καὶ
ὅστις ἐν μέθαις ἑταίραις τε καὶ κώμοις καταγίνεται.
τὸ δ' ἐπὶ μεγάλῃ βλάβῃ χρημάτων ἢ ἀτιμίᾳ μετρίως
ταραχθῆναι τὴν ψυχὴν οὐκέθ' ὁμοίως ἐστὶ φανερόν,
εἰ τοῦ γένους τῶν παθῶν ὑπάρχει, ὥσπερ οὐδὲ τὸ
πλακοῦντα φαγεῖν ἀκυρώτερον, ἀλλὰ καὶ ταῦτα
κατάδηλα γίνεται τῷ προμελετήσαντι τὴν ψυχὴν

great commandment.[16] I later saw that it is justly praised, for only the wisest might know himself accurately, but among all others none might do so accurately, though some do know themselves better or worse than others do. For just as in every aspect of life and in every craft, it is within everybody's power to recognize great achievements and distinctions in matters, but only knowledgeable and expert men can recognize the finer differences, so also this is true of errors $(5.9D = 5.5K)$ and affections. You clearly recognize that the sort of man who bites and kicks his staff when violently angry over trivial matters is in a state of affection, as is the sort of man who when drunk busies himself with escorts and parties. Being moderately troubled in spirit by a great financial loss or public disgrace falls less clearly into the category of affections (like eating cake immoderately does), but these [distinctions] are in fact obvious to someone who has

ἐξοδιάσαντί <τε> ἁπάντων παθῶν ἐπανορθώσεως δεόμενα·

ὅστις οὖν βούλεται καλὸς κἀγαθὸς γενέσθαι, τοῦτο ἐννοησάτω, ὡς ἀναγκαῖόν ἐστιν αὐτὸν ἀγνοεῖν πολλὰ τῶν ἰδίων ἁμαρτημάτων· ὅπως <δ'> ἂν ἐξεύροι πάντα, δυνάμενος ἐγὼ λέγειν, [ὅπ]ὡς εὑρὼν αὐτός, οὔπω λέγω, διότι τὸ βιβλίον τοῦτο δύναταί ποτε καὶ εἰς ἄλλων ἀφικέσθαι χεῖρας, ὅπως ἂν κἀκεῖνοι γυμνασθῶσι πρότερον ὁδὸν εὑρεῖν τῆς γνώσεως τῶν ἰδίων ἁμαρτημάτων. ὥσπερ <οὖν> καὶ σέ μοι λέγειν (5.23D = 5.6K) ἠξίωσα καί, μέχρι τὸ σαυτῷ δοκοῦν ἀπεφήνω, διεσιώπησα, καὶ νῦν οὕτω πράξω, παρακαλέσας τὸν ὁμιλοῦντα τῷδε τῷ γράμματι καταθέμενον αὐτὸ ζητῆσαι, ὅπως ἄν τις ἑαυτὸν δύναιτο [τὸ] γνωρίζειν ἁμαρτάνοντα.

trained his soul beforehand and has discharged what is necessary for the correction of all his affections.[17]

Therefore, whoever wants to become a fine and good person, let him bear this in mind, that one is necessarily unaware of many of one's own errors. How one could discover all of them, I am able to tell you, as I found out on my own, but I will not yet do so because this book at some point may come into the hands of other people, so that they, too, may first exert themselves to discover a method for recognizing their own personal errors. So, just as I thought it appropriate that you tell me [what you think] **(5.23D = 5.6K)** and remained silent for as long as you shared your opinions with me, now I will do the same: I ask the person who is joining in conversation with this text to set it aside and to examine how he might be able to recognize when he is committing an error.

δύο γάρ, ὡς Αἴσωπος ἔλεγε, πήρας ἐξήμμεθα τοῦ τραχήλου, τῶν μὲν ἀλλοτρίων τὴν πρόσω, τῶν ἰδίων δὲ τὴν ὀπίσω, καὶ διὰ τοῦτο τὰ μὲν ἀλλότρια βλέπομεν ἀεί, τῶν δ᾽ οἰκείων ἀθέατοι καθεστήκαμεν. καὶ τοῦτόν γε τὸν λόγον ὡς ἀληθῆ προσίενται πάντες. ὁ δὲ Πλάτων καὶ τὴν αἰτίαν ἀποδίδωσι τοῦ γιγνομένου· τυφλώττειν γάρ φησι τὸ φιλοῦν περὶ τὸ φιλούμενον. εἴπερ οὖν ἕκαστος ἡμῶν ἑαυτὸν ἁπάντων μάλιστα φιλεῖ, τυφλώττειν ἀναγκαῖόν ἐστιν αὐτὸν ἐφ᾽ ἑαυτοῦ. πῶς οὖν ὄψεται τὰ ἴδια κακά; καὶ πῶς ἁμαρτάνων γνώσεται; πολλῷ γὰρ ἔοικεν ὅ τε τοῦ Αἰσώπου μῦθος καὶ ὁ τοῦ Πλάτωνος λόγος ἀνελπιστοτέραν ἡμῖν τὴν τῶν ἰδίων ἁμαρτημάτων εὕρεσιν ἀποφαίνειν· εἰ γὰρ μὴ τοῦ φιλεῖν τις ἑαυτὸν ἀποστῆσαι δύναται, τυφλώττειν ἀναγκαῖόν ἐστι τὸ φιλοῦν περὶ τὸ φιλούμενον.

οὐ μὴν οὐδ᾽ ἐγὼ τὸν ἀναγινώσκοντα τόδε τὸ βιβλίον ἠξίουν ἂν **(6.17D = 5.7K)** ἐπισκέψασθαι καθ᾽

For we have, as Aesop said, two knapsacks around our necks, the one in front filled with the wrongs of others,[18] and the one in back with our own. Because of this, we are always able to see others' wrongs, but we are blind to our own. And everyone accepts this statement as true. Plato also provides the reason for this occurrence: he says that the lover is blind concerning the object of his love. If in fact each of us loves himself most of all, he is necessarily blind when it comes to himself. How, then, will he see his own wrongs? And how will he recognize when he errs? To many, Aesop's fable and Plato's argument seem to present our discovery of our personal errors as rather futile. For if someone is not able to set aside his love for himself, it is necessary that the lover be blind concerning the object of his love.

But I would not have considered my reader to be worthy of **(6.17D = 5.7K)** studying this

αὐτὸν <περὶ> τῆς τῶν ἰδίων ἁμαρτημάτων εὑρέσεως,
εἰ μὴ χαλεπὸν ἦν τὸ πρᾶγμα, κἄν τις ὡς ἐπὶ πλεῖστον ἐσκεμμένος ᾖ καθ' αὑτόν. καὶ τοίνυν ἐγὼ τὴν
ἐμὴν ἀποφαίνομαι γνώμην, ἵν', εἰ μέν τινα καὶ αὐτὸς
ἕκαστος ἑτέραν ὁδὸν εὕροι, προσλαβὼν καὶ τὴν ἐμὴν
ὠφεληθῇ πλέον ἅτε διπλῆν ἀνθ' ἁπλῆς εὑρὼν ὁδὸν
σωτηρίας· εἰ δὲ μή, ἀλλ' αὐτῇ γε τῇ ἡμετέρᾳ διατελῇ
χρώμενος, ἄχρι περ ἂν ἑτέραν εὕρῃ βελτίονα· τίς οὖν
ἡ ἐμή, λέγειν ἂν ἤδη καιρός, ἀρχὴν τῷ λόγῳ τήνδε
ποιησάμενον.

Ἐπειδὴ τὰ μὲν ἁμαρτήματα διὰ [τὴν] ψευδῆ δόξαν
γίγνονται, τὰ δὲ πάθη διά τιν' ἄλογον ὁρμήν, ἔδοξέ
μοι πρότερον ἑαυτὸν ἐλευθερῶσαι τῶν παθῶν· εἰκὸς
γάρ πως καὶ διὰ ταῦτα ψευδῶς ἡμᾶς δοξάζειν. ἔστι
δὲ πάθη ψυχῆς, ἅπερ ἅπαντες γινώσκουσι, θυμὸς καὶ
ὀργὴ καὶ φόβος καὶ λύπη καὶ φθόνος καὶ ἐπιθυμία

book for himself regarding the discovery of his own errors unless the matter were a difficult one, even for someone who was especially engaged in self-reflection. And now I am giving my own opinion, in order that, if each person should find any another method, he might be helped more by applying mine in addition, since he has discovered a double method for preserving himself instead of a single one. If not, at least he might continue using our method until he finds a better one. At this point, I will describe my approach, having already established the beginning of my argument.

Since on the one hand, errors are born of false beliefs, while affections are born of some irrational impulse, it seemed to me that one should first liberate himself from his affections, since it is likely that we somehow form false beliefs because of them. There are the affections of the soul that everyone knows: anger, rage, fear, grief,

σφοδρά. κατὰ δὲ τὴν ἐμὴν γνώμην καὶ τὸ φθάσαι πάνυ σφόδρα φιλεῖν ἢ μισεῖν ὁτιοῦν πρᾶγμα πάθος ἐστίν. ὀρθῶς γὰρ ἔοικεν εἰρῆσθαι τὸ "μέτρον ἄριστον", (7.6D = 5.8K) ὡς οὐδενὸς ἀμέτρου καλῶς γιγνομένου.

πῶς οὖν ἄν τις ἐκκόψειε ταῦτα μὴ γνοὺς πρότερον ἔχων αὐτά; γνῶναι δ᾽, ὡς ἐλέγομεν, ἀδύνατον, ἐπειδὴ σφόδρα φιλοῦμεν ἡμᾶς. ἀλλὰ κἂν μὴ σαυτὸν ὁ λόγος οὗτος ἐπιτρέπῃ σοι κρίνειν, ἄλλον γε συγχωρεῖ δύνασθαι κρῖναι τὸν μήτε φιλούμενον ὑπὸ σοῦ μήτε μισούμενον. ὅταν οὖν ἀκούσῃς τινὰ τῶν κατὰ τὴν πόλιν* ἐπαινούμενον ὑπὸ πολλῶν ἐπὶ τῷ μηδένα κολακεύειν, ἐκείνῳ προσφοιτήσας τῇ σαυτοῦ πείρᾳ κρῖνον, εἰ τοιοῦτός ἐστιν, οἷος εἶναι λέγεται, καὶ πρῶτον, ἐὰν ἴδῃς αὐτὸν ἐπὶ τὰς τῶν πλουσίων τε καὶ

---

* Omitting "ὃν μήτε φιλήσειν οἶδε μήτε <μισήσειν>," after De Boer, *Galeni De propriorum animi cuiuslibet affectuum dignotione et curatione*; and Singer, *Galen: Psychological Writings*.

envy, and violent desire. In addition, in my opinion, to swiftly form a violent feeling of love or hate for anything is also an affection. It seems to me that the phrase "moderation is best" is rightly stated, **(7.6D = 5.8K)** as no one does well without moderation.

So, how should someone eradicate these affections, if he from the start does not recognize that he has them? To recognize them, as we were saying, is impossible, since we love ourselves intensely. But although this argument does not leave it to you to judge yourself, it does on the other hand concede that it is possible to judge someone you neither love nor hate. So, whenever you hear that someone is praised throughout the city on the grounds that he does not flatter anybody, spend time with this man and, from your experience, judge for yourself if he is the sort of person he is said to be. First, if you

πολὺ δυναμένων ἢ καὶ τὰς τῶν μονάρχων οἰκίας
ἐπιόντα συνεχῶς, γίγνωσκε μάτην ἀκηκοέναι τὸν
ἄνθρωπον τοῦτον ἀληθεύειν ἅπαντα (ταῖς γὰρ
τοιαύταις κολακείαις ἕπεται καὶ τὸ ψεύδεσθαι), δεύτερον <ἢ προσαγορεύοντα> ἢ παραπέμποντα τοὺς
τοιούτους ὁρῶν αὐτὸν ἢ καὶ συνδειπνοῦντα. τοιοῦτον
γάρ τις ἑλόμενος βίον οὐ μόνον <οὐκ> ἀληθεύει,
(7.20D = 5.9K) ἀλλὰ καὶ κακίαν ὅλην ἐξ ἀνάγκης
ἔχει, φιλοχρήματος ὢν ἢ φίλαρχος ἢ φιλότιμος ἢ
φιλόδοξος, ἤ τινα τούτων ἢ πάντα.

τὸν δὲ μὴ προσαγορεύοντα μήτε παραπέμποντα
μήτε συνδειπνοῦντα τοῖς πολὺ δυναμένοις ἢ πλουτοῦσι καὶ κεκολασμένῃ τῇ διαίτῃ χρώμενον ἐλπίσας
ἀληθεύσειν εἰς βαθυτέραν ἀφικέσθαι πειρῶ γνῶσιν,
ὁποῖός τίς ἐστιν (ἐν συνουσίαις δ’ αὕτη πολυχρονιω-
τέραις γίγνεται), κἂν εὕρῃς τοιοῦτον, ἰδίᾳ ποτὲ

see him always going to the homes of the wealthy and powerful, or also at the houses of rulers, know that this man's reputation for always telling the truth is false, since lying also follows this kind of flattery. Second, this also holds true if you see him greeting, accompanying, or also dining with such people. Someone who chooses this kind of life not only does not tell the truth **(7.20D = 5.9K)** but also is necessarily thoroughly bad, since he will be some or all of these things: money loving, power grubbing, attention seeking, or image conscious.

On the other hand, if you entertain the hope that some man who does not greet, accompany, or dine with powerful or wealthy men and who enjoys a chastened lifestyle is truthful, try to come to a deeper understanding of what sort of man he is, as happens through an extended acquaintance. If you do find that he is truthful, ask

μόνῳ διαλέχθητι παρακαλέσας, ὅ τι ἂν <ἐν> σοὶ
βλέπῃ τῶν εἰρημένων παθῶν, εὐθέως δηλοῦν, ὡς
χάριν ἕξοντι τούτου μεγίστην ἡγησομένῳ τε σωτῆρα
μᾶλλον ἢ εἰ νοσοῦντα τὸ σῶμα διέσωσε. κἂν ὑπόσχη-
ται δηλώσειν, ὅταν ἴδῃ τι τῶν εἰρημένων πάσχοντά
σε, κἄπειτα πλειόνων ἡμερῶν μεταξὺ γιγνομένων
μηδὲν εἴπῃ συνδιατρίβων δηλονότι, μέμψαι τὸν ἄνθρωπον, αὖθίς τε παρακάλεσον ἔτι λιπαρέστερον ἢ
ὡς πρόσθεν, ὅ τι ἂν ὑπὸ σοῦ βλέπῃ κατὰ πάθος
πραττόμενον, εὐθέως μηνύειν. ἐὰν δ' εἴπῃ σοι, διὰ
τὸ μηδὲν ἑωρακέναι περὶ σὲ τοιοῦτον ἐν τῷ μεταξύ,
διὰ τοῦτο μηδ' αὐτὸς εἰρηκέναι, μὴ πεισθῇς
(8.11D = 5.10K) εὐθέως μηδ' οἰηθῇς ἀναμάρτητος
ἐξαίφνης γεγονέναι, ἀλλὰ δυοῖν θάτερον, ἢ διὰ ῥαθυ-
μίαν οὐ προσεσχηκέναι σοι τὸν παρακληθέντα

to speak with him alone in private, and then ask that, if he should see any of these affections in you, he disclose them frankly to you. Tell him that you would be most grateful to him, even more than if he saved your body when it was sick. Then, if he does take it upon himself to point out to you whenever he sees you suffering from any of the aforementioned affections, and then after having spent time with you for a few days in the meantime still provides no clear feedback, reprimand him and ask him again—even more earnestly than before—to frankly reveal whatever he sees you do under the influence of an affection. If he tells you that he has said nothing because he has not seen any such thing from you in this time period, do not be so quick to trust him, and **(8.11D = 5.10K)** do not think that you have suddenly become perfect. Instead, consider one of two options: either the friend you called upon is not paying close

φίλον ἢ ἐλέγχειν αἰδούμενον σιωπᾶν ἢ καὶ μισηθῆ-
ναι μὴ βουλόμενον διὰ τὸ γινώσκειν ἅπασιν ὡς ἔπος
εἰπεῖν ἀνθρώποις ἔθος εἶναι μισεῖν τοὺς τἀληθῆ λέ-
γοντας, ἢ εἰ μὴ διὰ ταῦτα, ἴσως <μὴ> βουλόμενον
αὐτὸν ὠφελεῖν σε διὰ τοῦτο σιωπᾶν, ἢ καὶ <δι᾽>
ἄλλην τινὰ [ἴσως] αἰτίαν, ἣν οὐκ ἐπαινοῦμεν ἡμεῖς.
ἀδύνατον γὰρ εἶναι τὸ μηδὲν ἡμαρτῆσθαί σοι, πιστεύ-
σας ἐμοὶ τοῦτο νῦν ἐπαινέσεις <μ᾽> ὕστερον, θεώμε-
νος ἅπαντας ἀνθρώπους καθ᾽ ἑκάστην ἡμέραν μυρία
μὲν ἁμαρτάνοντας καὶ κατὰ πάθος πράττοντας, οὐ
μὴν αὐτούς γε παρακολουθοῦντας. ὥστε μηδὲ σὺ νόμιζε σαυτὸν ἄλλο τι καὶ μὴ ἄνθρωπον εἶναι. νομίζεις
δ᾽ ἄλλο τι μᾶλλον <ἢ> ἄνθρωπος ὑπάρχειν, ἐὰν ἀνα-
πείσῃς σαυτὸν ἅπαντα καλῶς σοι πεπρᾶχθαι μὴ ὅτι
μηνὸς ἑνός, ἀλλὰ μιᾶς ἡμέρας.

ἴσως οὖν ἐρεῖς, <ἢν> ἀντιλογικὸς ᾖς, ἤτοι κατὰ
προαίρεσιν ἢ ἐκ (9.4D = 5.11K) μοχθηροῦ τινος ἔθους
γεγονὼς τοιοῦτος ἢ καὶ φύσει φιλόνεικος ὤν, ὅσον

attention to you owing to laziness, or he is silent because he is ashamed to correct you or does not want you to hate him, since he knows that practically all men hate those who tell the truth. If it is none of these reasons, it could also be that he is quiet because he does not want to help you, or for some other reason that is not praiseworthy. For it is impossible that you made no error—trust me on this now, and you will praise me later—when you see that everyone daily makes countless errors and acts under the influence of affections without paying attention to what they are doing. So do not think that you are something other than human—as you are in fact doing if you cling to the idea that you have done everything well for a whole month, or even for a single day.

If you are a contrarian, because you choose to be, because you have developed into one because of **(9.4D = 5.11K)** a character flaw, or

ἐπὶ τῷ νῦν ὑπ᾽ ἐμοῦ προκεχειρισμένῳ λόγῳ, τοὺς σο-
φοὺς ἄνδρας ἄλλο τι μᾶλλον ἢ ἀνθρώπους εἶναι.
τούτῳ δή σου τῷ λόγῳ τὸν ἡμέτερον ἀντίθες διττὸν
ὄντα, τὸν μὲν ἕτερον, ὅτι μόνος ὁ σοφὸς ἀναμάρτητός
ἐστι τὸ πάμπαν, ἕτερον δ᾽ ἐπ᾽ αὐτῷ τῷ προϊεμένῳ,
εἴπερ ἀναμάρτητός ἐστιν ὁ σοφός, οὐδ᾽ ἄνθρωπον
ὑπάρχειν αὐτὸν ὅσον ἐπὶ τῷδε. καὶ διὰ τοῦτο τῶν
παλαιοτάτων φιλοσόφων ἀκούσῃ λεγόντων ὁμοίω-
σιν εἶναι θεῷ τὴν σοφίαν. ἀλλὰ σύ γε θεῷ παραπλή-
σιος ἐξαίφνης οὐκ ἄν ποτε γένοιο. ὅπου γὰρ οἱ δι᾽
ὅλου τοῦ βίου <τὴν> ἀπάθειαν ἀσκήσαντες οὐ πι-
στεύονται τελέως αὐτὴν ἐσχηκέναι, πολὺ δήπου μᾶλλον ὁ μηδέποτ᾽ ἀσκήσας σύ· μὴ τοίνυν πιστεύσῃς τῷ
λέγοντι μηδὲν ἑωρακέναι κατὰ πάθος ὑπὸ σοῦ πραττόμενον, ἀλλ᾽ ἤτοι μὴ βουλόμενον ὠφελεῖν σε νόμιζε

because you are just quarrelsome by nature, then you will say that, according to the argument I am making, wise men are something other than human. Set my two-part reply against this argument of yours: first, only the wise man is completely without error. Second, in response to your utterance that, "if a wise man is without error, then he is not even a man to the extent he is in this condition," it is in fact because of this that you will hear the most ancient philosophers say that attaining wisdom is like becoming a god. But you cannot become god-like immediately. For if those who have trained their whole lives to be free from affections are unsure that they have achieved this state in the end, how much the more does this apply to you, having never (I presume) undertaken such training. You should therefore not trust the man who tells you that he has never seen you do anything under the influence of an affection.

λέγειν οὕτως, ἢ μὴ παραφυλάξαι προηρημένον, ἃ πράττεις κακῶς, ἢ φυλαττόμενον ὑπὸ σοῦ μισηθῆναι· τάχα δὲ καὶ εἶδέ σέ ποτε δυσχεράναντα πρὸς τὸν ἐπιτιμήσαντα τοῖς σοῖς ἁμαρτήμασί τε (9.19D = 5.12K) καὶ πάθεσι, ὥστ' εἰκότως σιωπᾷ, μὴ πιστεύων ἀληθεύειν σε λέγοντα βούλεσθαι ἕκαστον εἰδέναι, ὧν ἁμαρτάνεις. ἐὰν δὲ <τὸ> πρῶτον τῶν ὑπὸ σοῦ <κατὰ πάθος> πραττομένων ἀπαλλαγεὶς σιωπήσῃς, εὑρήσεις πολλοὺς ὀλίγον ὕστερον ἀληθῶς ἐπανορθουμένους σε, καὶ πόλυ γε μᾶλλον, ἐὰν χάριν γνῷς τῷ μεμψαμένῳ χωρισθείσης σου τῆς βλάβης τούτου γ' ἕνεκεν. ἐξ αὐτοῦ δὲ τοῦ διασκέψασθαι, πότερον ἀληθῶς ἢ ψευδῶς ἐπετίμησέ σοι, μεγάλης ὠφελείας αἰσθήσῃ, κἂν συνεχῶς πράττῃς αὐτὸ προηρημένος ὄντως εἷς γενέσθαι καλὸς κἀγαθός, ἔσῃ τοιοῦτος.

Instead, you should think that he said this because he does not want to help you, or that he deliberately chose not to keep a close eye on what you did wrongly, or that he is trying to guard against your hatred. Perhaps he even once saw you get annoyed at someone who was censuring your errors **(9.19D = 5.12K)** and affections, so that he is reasonably silent because he does not trust that you tell the truth when you say that you want him to know each error that you make. But if first you free yourself from such actions undertaken in affection and keep silent, you will find that, in a little while, many will correct you honestly. They will do so even more if you make known your gratitude to the one correcting you, because he has separated you from harm. And from this careful evaluation of whether he censured you truly or falsely, you will perceive a tremendous benefit for yourself, and if you do this continually, really

ἐν μὲν δὴ τῷ πρώτῳ χρόνῳ μηδ᾽ ἐὰν καὶ σκεπτό-
μενος ἀκριβῶς εὕρῃς ἐπηρεαστικῶς τε καὶ ψευδῶς
[ὡς] ἐγκεκληκότα σοί τινα, πειρῶ σαυτὸν πείθειν, ὡς
οὐδὲν ἥμαρτες, ἀλλά σοι τοῦτο πρῶτον φιλοσό-
φημα τὸ καρτερεῖν ἐπηρεαζόμενον. ὕστερον δέ ποτε
κατεσταλμένων ἱκανῶς <τῶν> σαυτοῦ παθῶν αἰσθό-
μενος ἐπιχειρήσεις ἀπολογεῖσθαι τοῖς ἐπηρεάζουσι
μηδέποτε πικρῶς μηδ᾽ ἐλεγκτικῶς μηδέ τοι φιλόνει-
κως ἐμφαίνων [μηδὲ] καταβάλλειν ἐθέλειν ἐκεῖνον,
ἀλλ᾽ ὠφελείας ἕνεκα τῆς σῆς, ἵνα τι καὶ πρὸς
τὴν ἀντιλογίαν ἀντειπόντος αὐτοῦ πιθανὸν ἤτοι
(10.13D = 5.13K) πεισθῇς ἐκεῖνον ἄμεινον γιγνώσκειν ἢ μετὰ πλείονος ἐξετάσεως εὕρῃς αὐτὸν ἔξω
τῶν ἐγκλημάτων <ὄντα>. Οὕτω γοῦν καὶ Ζήνων
ἠξίου πάντα πράττειν ἡμᾶς ἀσφαλῶς, ὡς ἀπολο-
γησαμένους ὀλίγον <ὕστερον τοῖς παιδαγωγοῖς>.

choosing to become a fine and good person, you will become one.

In the early period of your evaluation, even if you have found after exacting examination that someone has accused you insolently and falsely, do not try to convince yourself that you have not erred, but keep as your first rule of conduct forbearance of insult. Later, when you perceive that your affections have been appropriately restrained, you will try to speak in defense of yourself against those who insult you, making clear that you do not wish to abuse this person in a bitter, adversarial, or contentious way, but rather that you are responding for the sake of your own benefit, either so that **(10.13D = 5.13K)** you may be persuaded that your opponent knows better if he presents a credible counterargument to your response, or so that, with greater scrutiny, you will find that he is without grounds for complaint. In this way

ὠνόμαζε γὰρ οὕτως ἐκεῖνος ὁ ἀνὴρ τοὺς πολλοὺς τῶν ἀνθρώπων ἑτοίμους ὄντας τοῖς πέλας ἐπιτιμᾶν, κἂν μηδεὶς αὐτοὺς παρακαλῇ.

Χρὴ δὲ τὸν ἀκούοντα μήτε πλούσιον εἶναι μήτε αἰ-δοῦς ἔχειν πολιτικῆς, ὡς, ἄν γε ταύτην ἔχῃ, διὰ φόβον οὐδεὶς αὐτῷ τἀληθῆ λέξει, καθάπερ οὐδὲ τοῖς πλουτοῦσι διὰ κέρδος οἱ κόλακες· ἀλλὰ κἂν εἴ τις ἀληθεύων παραφανῇ, διανίσταται πρὸς αὐτῶν. ἐὰν οὖν τις ἤτοι πολλὰ δυνάμενος ἢ καὶ πλούσιος ἐθελήσῃ γενέσθαι καλὸς κἀγαθός, ἀποθέσθαι πρότερον αὐτὸν δεήσει ταῦτα, καὶ μάλιστα νῦν, ὅπου <γ'> οὐχ εὑρή-σει Διογένη δυνάμενον εἰπεῖν τούτῳ τἀληθῆ, κἂν πλουσιώτατος ᾖ, κἂν μόναρχος.

Zeno in fact believed that we should do everything steadfastly, as if we were to defend these actions to our teachers a little later—and "teachers" is what he named the mass of men who are ready to rebuke the people around them, even if no one asks them for their opinion.

The person listening to such criticism must neither be rich nor cling to the politician's political ambition.[19] In the latter case, no one will speak the truth to him, because of fear, but in the former case, flatterers do not want to tell the truth to rich men because of desire for monetary gain. But, if someone demonstrates that he tells the truth, he is distinguished from these other types. And if someone powerful or wealthy wants to become a good and honest man, he first needs to disregard his wealth and power, especially so today, when he will not be able to find anywhere a Diogenes who can tell him the truth—especially if he is very wealthy or a king.

ἐκεῖνοι μὲν οὖν ὑπὲρ ἑαυτῶν βουλεύσονται· σὺ δ' ὁ μὴ πλούσιος μηδὲ δυνατὸς ἐν πόλει πᾶσι μὲν ἐπίτρεπε λέγειν, ἃ καταγινώσκουσί σου, πρὸς μηδένα δ' αὐτὸς ἀγανάκτει, καὶ οὕτως ἔχε πάντας, ὡς **(11.7D = 5.14K)** Ζήνων ἔλεγε, παιδαγωγούς. οὐ μὴν ὁμοίως σε πᾶσι περὶ ὧν ἂν εἴπωσιν ἀξιῶ προσέχειν, ἀλλὰ τοῖς ἄριστα βεβιωκόσι πρεσβύταις. ὁποῖοι δ' εἰσὶν οἱ ἄριστα βιοῦντες, ὀλίγον ἔμπροσθεν εἶπον. ἐν δὲ τῷ χρόνῳ προϊόντι καὶ χωρὶς ἐκείνων αὐτὸς παρακολουθήσεις καὶ γνώσῃ, πηλίκα πρόσθεν [ἦν, ἄν] ἥμαρτες, ἡνίκα μάλιστα ἐγώ σοι φανοῦμαι λέγων τἀληθῆ, μηδένα φάσκων ἔξω παθῶν ἢ ἁμαρτημάτων εἶναι, μηδ' ἂν εὐφυέστατος ᾖ, μηδ' ἂν <ἐν> ἔθεσι καλλίστοις τεθραμμένος, ἀλλὰ πάντως τινὰ σφάλλεσθαι καὶ μᾶλλον, ὅταν ἔτι νέος ᾖ.

These sorts of people will deliberate on their own behalf, but you, who are neither rich nor powerful in the city, entrust it to everyone in the city to tell you what they observe about you, and do not be angry with any of them, and regard them all, as **(11.7D = 5.14K)** Zeno said, as your teachers. Not that I think you should consider what everyone says to be of equal value, but rather you should pay special attention to older men who have lived the best sorts of lives. (I previously described the kinds of men who live the best lives.) With the passage of time, even without them you will pay close attention and recognize the magnitude of your previous errors. Then, you will really acknowledge that I told you the truth when I said that no one is without affections or errors, not even the person of the naturally best disposition who was raised with the finest habits,

Δεῖται γὰρ ἀσκήσεως ἕκαστος ἡμῶν σχεδὸν <δι'> ὅλου τοῦ βίου πρὸς τὸ γενέσθαι τέλειος ἀνήρ. οὐ μὴν ἀφίστασθαι χρὴ τοῦ βελτίω ποιεῖν ἑαυτόν, εἰ καὶ πεντηκοντούτης τις ὢν αἴσθοιτο τὴν ψυχὴν λελωβημένος οὐκ ἀνίατον οὐδ' ἀνεπανόρθωτον λώβην. οὐδὲ γὰρ εἰ τὸ σῶμα κακῶς διέκειτο πεντηκοντούτης ὤν, ἔκδοτον ἂν ἔδωκε τῇ (11.20D = 5.15K) καχεξίᾳ, πάντως <δ'> ἂν ἐπειράθη βέλτιον αὐτὸ κατασκευάσαι, καίτοι τὴν Ἡράκλειον εὐεξίαν οὐ δυνάμενος σχεῖν. μὴ τοίνυν μηδ' ἡμεῖς ἀφιστώμεθα τοῦ βελτίω τὴν ψυχὴν ἐργάζεσθαι, κἂν τὴν τοῦ σοφοῦ μὴ δυνώμεθα σχεῖν, ἀλλὰ μάλιστα μὲν ἐλπίζωμεν ἕξειν κἀκείνην, ἂν ἐκ μειρακίου προνοώμεθα τῆς ψυχῆς ἡμῶν, εἰ δὲ μή, ἀλλὰ τοῦ γε μὴ πάναισχρον αὐτὴν γενέσθαι, καθάπερ ὁ Θερσίτης τὸ σῶμα, φροντίζωμεν.

but truly everyone makes mistakes, and all the more when they are young.

Becoming a perfect person necessitates training in each of us more or less throughout one's whole life. One should not give up on trying to make oneself better, even if fifty years old, if one perceives an imperfection in one's soul that is not incurable or irreparable. For if one were in a bad condition in body at fifty years old, one would not simply abandon **(1L.20D = 5.15K)** the body to the poor condition, but instead would endeavor to improve it in every way, even if he could not acquire the fine condition of Hercules. So then, let us not be deterred from working to improve the soul. And if we are unable to acquire the condition of the wise man, let us aspire to it as much as we can and be attentive to our souls from our adolescence, or otherwise let us at least take care that it not become totally ugly, like the body of Thersites.[20]

Prognosis, for Epigenes

Addressed to a friend (Epigenes), this text describes Galen's first few years in Rome as a young physician. Richly narrated, "Prognosis, for Epigenes" records multiple encounters with patients, as well as Galen's confrontations with physicians who challenged his theories and methods. Galen also emphasizes the importance of prognosing, or predicting, the course of disease and discusses how he is able to make accurate prognoses based on his powers of observation

and knowledge of anatomy and physiology. Here, he records a case history of one of the patients he treated during this period, emphasizing his own incisive powers of observation (especially in the case of a reticent patient), his knowledge of the pulse, and his links with other celebrated physicians of the past. The text emphasizes what we all know from personal experience and what is increasingly being demonstrated on a biomolecular level, namely that our mental state affects our physical condition.

(14.631.5K) Παρεκλήθην μὲν εἰς τὴν ἐπίσκεψιν τῆς γυναικὸς ὡς ἀγρυπνούσης ἐν ταῖς νυξὶ καὶ μεταβαλλούσης ἑαυτὴν ἄλλοτ᾽ εἰς ἄλλο σχῆμα κατακλίσεως, εὑρὼν δ᾽ ἀπύρετον ἐπυθόμην ὑπὲρ ἑκάστου τῶν κατὰ μέρος αὐτῇ γεγονότων ἐξ ὧν ἴσμεν ἀγρυπνίας συμβαινούσας. ἡ δὲ μόγις ἢ οὐδ᾽ ὅλως ἀπεκρίνετο, ὡς μάτην ἐρωτωμένην ἐνδεικνυμένη[ν], καὶ τὸ τελευταῖον ἀποστραφεῖσα τοῖς μὲν ἐπιβεβλημένοις ἱματίοις ὅλῳ τῷ σώματι σκεπάσασα πᾶσαν ἑαυτὴν ἄλλῳ δε τινι μικρῷ ταραντινιδίῳ τὴν κεφαλὴν ἔκειτο καθάπερ οἱ χρῄζοντες ὕπνου.

Χωρισθεὶς οὖν ἐγὼ δυοῖν θάτερον αὐτὴν ἐνόησα πάσχειν, ἢ μελαγχολικῶς δυσθυμεῖν ἤ τι λυπουμένην οὐκ ἐθέλειν ὁμολογεῖν. Εἰς τὴν ὑστεραίαν οὖν ἀνεβαλ[λ]όμην ἀκριβέστερον διασκέψασθαι περὶ

PHYSIOLOGICAL CONSEQUENCES
OF UNREQUITED LOVE

(14.631.5K) I was called to examine a woman who had spent many sleepless nights tossing and turning in bed. Finding her to be afebrile, I asked her what might have happened to different parts of her body, from which we know insomnia occurs. She either answered me with great effort or said absolutely nothing, as if showing that it was pointless to ask these questions. Finally, she turned her back to me, covering her whole body with piles of blankets and her head with a small cloth wrap, and lay there like those who want to sleep.

After I left, I thought that she suffered from one of two problems: either she was depressed on account of black bile,[21] or she was pained in some way that she did not want to admit. So, I delayed a more detailed questioning of her until

(14.632K) αὐτῶν καὶ πορευθεὶς τὸ μὲν πρῶτον ἤκουσα τῆς παραμενούσης οἰκέτιδος ὡς ἀδύνατον αὐτὴν ἄρτι θεάσασθαι· δεύτερον δ'ἐπανελθὼν ὡς ἤκουσα πάλιν ταὐτό, τρίτον αὖθις ἦκον. εἰπούσης δέ μοι τῆς θεραπαίνης ἀπαλλάττεσθαι, μὴ βούλεσθαι γὰρ ἐνοχλεῖσθαι τὴν γυναῖκα, καὶ γνοὺς αὐτὴν ἐμοῦ χωρισθέντος λελουμένην τε καὶ τῶν συνηθῶν προσενηνεγμένην ἦκον τῇ ὑστεραίᾳ καὶ μόνος διαλεχθεὶς τῇ θεραπαίνῃ πολυειδῶς, ἔγνων σαφῶς τινι λύπῃ τειρομένην, ἣν ἐξεῦρον κατὰ τύχην, ὁποίαν οἶμαι καὶ Ἐρασιστράτῳ γενέσθαι. προεγνωσμένου γάρ μοι τοῦ μηδὲν εἶναι κατὰ τὸ σῶμα πάθος ἀλλ᾽ ἀπὸ ψυχικῆς τινος ἀηδίας ἐνοχλεῖσθαι τὴν γυναῖκα συνέβη κατὰ τὸν αὐτὸν καιρὸν ὃν ἐπεσκόπουν αὐτὴν βεβαιωθῆναι τοῦτο παραγενομένου τινὸς ἐκ τοῦ θεάτρου καὶ φάντος ὀρχούμενον ἑωρακέναι Πυλάδην· ἠλλάγη γὰρ

the next day. **(14.632K)** When I arrived for the first time, I heard from her maidservant that it was not possible to see her at that moment. Returning a second time, I heard the same thing again. Then I came a third time, and the maidservant told me to leave, saying that the woman did not want to be bothered. Learning that she had taken her bath and eaten as usual, I visited on the following day and chatted alone with her maidservant about a variety of topics and learned that the woman was beset by some grief—something I found out by pure luck, as I think Erasistratus also did.[22] And after I determined that she did not have anything physically wrong with her but that she was disturbed by some psychological distress, it happened that this was confirmed right on the same occasion when I had come to see her, when someone who had come from the theater said that he had seen Pylades dancing. Her eyes and the complexion

αὐτῆς καὶ τὸ βλέμμα καὶ τὸ χρῶμα τοῦ προσώπου, κἀγὼ θεασάμενος τοῦτο, τῷ καρπῷ τῆς γυναικὸς ἐπιβαλὼν τὴν χεῖρα, τὸν σφυγμὸν εὗρον ἀνώμαλον ἐξαίφνης πολυειδῶς γενόμενον, ὅστις δηλοῖ τὴν ψυχὴν τεθορυβῆσθαι· ὁ αὐτὸς οὖν καὶ τοῖς ἀγωνιῶσι περί τι πρᾶγμα (14.633K) συμβαίνειν. κατὰ τὴν ὑστεραίαν οὖν εἰπὼν ἀκολούθῳ τινὶ τῶν ἐμῶν, ὅταν ἐπισκεψάμενος ἔλθω πρὸς τὴν γυναῖκα, μετ᾽ ὀλίγον ἀφικόμενος ἀνάγγειλαί μοι, Μόρφον ὀρχεῖσθαι τήμερον, εἶθ᾽ ὡς ἤγγειλεν, ἄτρεπτον εὗρον τὸν σφυγμόν. ὁμοίως δὲ καὶ κατὰ τὴν ἑξῆς ἡμέραν ποιήσας ἀγγελθῆναι περὶ τοῦ τρίτου τῶν ὀρχηστῶν, ὁμοίως μείναντος ἀτρέπτου τοῦ σφυγμοῦ, κατὰ τὴν τετάρτην ἠκρίβωσα νύκτα πάνυ παραφυλάξας, ἡνίκα Πυλάδης ὀρχούμενος ἠγγέλθη παραχρῆμα ταραχθέντα πολυειδῶς ἰδὼν αὐτὸν εὗρον οὕτως ἐρῶσαν τοῦ Πυλάδου τὴν γυναῖκα καὶ τοῦτο παραφυλαχθὲν

of her face completely changed, and when I noticed this, I put my hand on her wrist and found that her pulse had immediately become irregular with respect to several metrics, making clear that her soul was disturbed. The same pulse is also found in those who are competing for something. **(14.633K)** The next day, I said to one of those who accompanied me on my rounds that once I had come to examine the woman, he should arrive a little after I did and report to me that Morphus was dancing today. When he made the announcement, I found that her pulse was unchanged. Similarly, on the following day, when my attendant reported on a third member of the dancing group, her pulse again remained undisturbed. But on the fourth night, I paid very close attention, and when it was reported that Pylades was dancing, I saw that her pulse immediately became very irregularly disturbed and so discovered that the woman was

ἀκριβῶς ἐν ταῖς ἐφεξῆς ἡμέραις εὑρέθη βεβαίως,
καθάπερ γε καί τινος ἄλλου τῶν πλουσίων δοῦλος
οἰκονόμος ὁμοίως κάμνων ἐγνώσθη μοι.

in love with Pylades. I carefully observed this and in the coming days ascertained it fully, just as indeed I learned that the enslaved household manager of some other rich person suffered from the same condition.

2

Exercising the Body

Age-appropriate physical activity was an essential part of maintaining health, although Galen was adamant that the excessive exercise of high-level athletes was ill advised and even dangerous. As an example of someone who exercises in an age-appropriate way, Galen mentions the Roman physician Antiochus, who in his eighties would make his daily rounds to see patients on foot; he would be carried on a litter or travel on a chariot only if the distance was more than was suitable for walking. Exercises of varying intensity and duration (all of which can be done without much, if any, equipment) are described in fascinating detail and (most) would still be

just as helpful for promoting strength and mobility as they ever were.

On Exercise with a Small Ball

In this charming short work, which I have included in its entirety, Galen describes what he calls the ideal exercise, one that involves mental activity, movement of all parts of the body, and the possibility of engaging in the activity alongside others. It is difficult to know precisely what this game looked like or entailed; for additional literature about ancient exercise, see "Further Reading" at the end of this book. There is the amusing possibility that Galen is being a bit tongue-in-cheek here by providing, with great

rhetorical flourish, an elevated description of a simple game, although it is also plausible that he did, indeed, intend for his detailed assessment of this exercise to be taken very seriously. Elsewhere in his work (including in the next passage I have provided), he describes other beneficial exercises, so he does not seem to have considered "the exercise with a small ball" to be the only activity beneficial for health. If Galen is in fact being serious in his praise of the benefits of this exercise, then his focus on its efficiency (you can exercise the upper and lower body at once!) does indeed sound like a modern way to tout a fitness regimen.

(1 = 5.899K) Πηλίκον μὲν ἀγαθόν ἐστιν, <ὦ Ἐπίγε-
νες,> εἰς ὑγίειαν γυμνάσια, καὶ ὡς χρὴ τῶν σιτίων
ἡγεῖσθαι αὐτά, παλαιοῖς ἀνδράσιν αὐτάρκως εἴρηται,
φιλοσόφων τε καὶ ἰατρῶν τοῖς ἀρίστοις· ὅσον δ᾽ ὑπὲρ
τἄλλα τὰ διὰ τῆς σμικρᾶς σφαίρας ἐστί, τοῦτ᾽ οὐ-
δέπω τῶν πρόσθεν ἱκανῶς οὐδεὶς ἐξηγήσατο. δίκαιον
οὖν ἡμᾶς ἃ γιγνώσκομεν εἰπεῖν, ὑπὸ σοῦ μὲν κριθη-
σόμενα τοῦ πάντων ἠσκηκότος ἄριστα τὴν ἐν αὐτοῖς
τέχνην, χρήσιμα δ᾽,<εἴπερ> ἱκανῶς εἰρῆσθαι δό-
ξειε, καὶ τοῖς ἄλλοις, οἷς ἂν μεταδῷς τοῦ λόγου,
γενησόμενα.

φημὶ γὰρ ἄριστα μὲν ἁπάντων γυμνασίων εἶναι τὰ
μὴ μόνον (5.900K) τὸ σῶμα διαπονεῖν, ἀλλὰ καὶ τὴν
ψυχὴν τέρπειν δυνάμενα. καὶ ὅσοι κυνηγέσια καὶ

THE IDEAL WORKOUT FOR HEALTH
AND WELLNESS

(1 = 5.899K) How great a good, Epigenes, physical exercise is for health, and how it ought to take precedence over food, was adequately stated by men of earlier generations, the best philosophers as well as doctors. But how much greater the exercise with the small ball is than other exercises no one of those before has ever sufficiently expounded. So it is right for us to say what we know, not only so that these things may be evaluated by you, who are most practiced in the art in this field, but also so that they may be useful, if they should seem sufficiently stated, also for whomever else you might share this treatise with.

I claim that the best of all exercises are those that have the capacity not only **(5.900K)** to train the body but also to delight the soul. The men

τὴν ἄλλην θήραν ἐξεῦρον, ἡδονῇ καὶ τέρψει καὶ φιλοτιμίᾳ τὸν ἐν αὐτοῖς πόνον κερασάμενοι, σοφοί τινες
ἄνδρες ἦσαν καὶ φύσιν ἀνθρωπίνην ἀκριβῶς κατα-
μεμαθηκότες. τοσοῦτον γὰρ ἐν αὐτῇ δύναται ψυχῆς
κίνησις, ὥστε πολλοὶ μὲν ἀπηλλάγησαν νοσημάτων
ἡσθέντες μόνον, πολλοὶ δ᾽ ἑάλωσαν ἀνιαθέντες. οὐδ᾽
ἔστιν οὐδὲν οὕτως ἰσχυρόν τι τῶν κατὰ τὸ σῶμα πα-
θημάτων, ὡς κρατεῖν τῶν περὶ τὴν ψυχήν. οὔκουν
οὐδ᾽ ἀμελεῖν χρὴ τῶν ταύτης κινήσεων ὁποῖαί τινες
ἔσονται, πολὺ δὲ μᾶλλον ἢ τῶν τοῦ σώματος ἐπιμε-
λεῖσθαι τά τ᾽ ἄλλα καὶ ὅσῳ κυριώτεραι. τοῦτο μὲν
δὴ κοινὸν ἁπάντων γυμνασίων τῶν μετὰ τέρψεως,
ἄλλα δ᾽ ἐξαίρετα τῶν διὰ τῆς σμικρᾶς σφαίρας, ἃ ἐγὼ
νῦν ἐξηγήσομαι.

who discovered dog hunting and other kinds of hunting, tempering the exertion of these activities with pleasure, joy, and ambitious rivalry, were wise and had a precise understanding of human nature. For the movement of the soul in this [activity] is so powerful that many have been delivered from sickness simply by the experience of pleasure, while many others have succumbed by the experience of grief. There is no kind of affection of the body so strong that it can overpower those concerning the soul. Hence, we must not disregard what kind of movements the soul will undergo either, but rather attend to them much more closely than those of the body, especially insofar as they are the more important. This indeed is common to all exercises that are accompanied by pleasure, but the exercise with the small ball is singular, as I will now describe.

(2) Πρῶτον μὲν ἡ εὐπορία. εἰ γοῦν ἐννοήσειας, ὅσης δεῖται παρασκευῆς θ' ἅμα καὶ σχολῆς τά τ' ἄλλα πάντα τὰ περὶ θήραν ἐπιτηδεύματα καὶ τὰ κυνηγέσια, (5.901K) σαφῶς ἂν μάθοις, ὡς οὔτε τῶν τὰ πολιτικὰ πραττόντων οὐδεὶς οὔτε τῶν τὰς τέχνας ἐργαζομένων δυνατὸς μεταχειρίζεσθαι τὰ τοιαῦτα γυμνάσια. καὶ γὰρ πλουτοῦντος δεῖται πολλῶν καὶ σχολὴν ἄγοντος οὐκ ὀλίγην ἀνθρώπου. τοῦτο δὲ μόνον οὕτω μὲν φιλάνθρωπον, ὡς μηδὲ τὸν πενέστατον ἀπορεῖν τῆς ἐπ' αὐτὸ παρασκευῆς (οὐ γὰρ δικτύων οὐδ' ὅπλων οὐδ' ἵππων οὐδὲ κυνῶν θηρευτικῶν, ἀλλὰ σφαίρας μόνης δεῖται καὶ ταύτης σμικρᾶς), οὕτω δ' εὔγνωμον εἰς τὰς ἄλλας πράξεις, ὥστ' οὐδεμιᾶς αὐτῶν ὀλιγωρεῖν ἀναγκάζει δι' αὐτό. καίτοι τί ἂν εὐπορώτερον γένοιτο τοῦ καὶ τύχην ἀνθρωπίνην ἅπασαν καὶ πρᾶξιν προσιεμένου; τῶν μὲν γὰρ ἀμφὶ τὰς

(2) First, there is convenience. If you keep in mind how much equipment and leisure time all the other hunting practices and hunting with dogs require, (5.901K) then you would clearly understand that no one who is involved in politics or engaged in the arts can participate in such kinds of exercises. For they require that a man be very wealthy and have no little leisure time. But exercising with the small ball is so generously available to everyone that not even the poorest man lacks the equipment for it, since it does not require nets, arms, horses, or hunting dogs—only a ball, and a small one at that. It is so considerate of other activities that it compels no one to neglect any of them on its account. And what could be more accessible than that which admits those of every human social class and activity? Enjoyment of exercises in the hunt is not easily accessible, since hunting requires wealth for the provision of the

θήρας γυμνασίων τῆς χρήσεως οὐκ ἐφ᾽ ἡμῖν ἡ εὐ-
πορία· πλούτου τε γὰρ δεῖται τὴν παρασκευὴν τῶν
ὀργάνων ἐκπορίζοντος καὶ ἀργίας σχολῇ τὸν καιρὸν
ἐπιτηρούσης. τούτου δ᾽ ἡ τῶν ὀργάνων παρασκευὴ
καὶ τοῖς πενεστάτοις εὔπορος, ὅ τε καιρὸς τῆς χρήσεως καὶ τοὺς ἱκανῶς ἀσχόλους ἀναμένει. τὸ μὲν δὴ
τῆς εὐπορίας αὐτοῦ τηλικοῦτον ἀγαθόν.

ὅτι δὲ καὶ πολυαρκέστατον τῶν ἄλλων (5.902K)
γυμνασίων, ὧδ᾽ ἂν μάλιστα μάθοις, εἰ σκέψαιο καθ᾽
ἕκαστον αὐτῶν, ὅ τί τε δύναται καὶ οἷόν τι τὴν φύσιν
ἐστίν. εὑρήσεις γὰρ ἢ σφοδρὸν ἢ μαλακὸν ἢ τὰ κάτω
μᾶλλον ἢ τὰ ἄνω κινοῦν ἢ μέρος τι πρὸ τῶν ἄλλων,
οἷον ὀσφὺν ἢ κεφαλὴν ἢ χεῖρας ἢ θώρακα, πάντα δ᾽
ἐξ ἴσου τὰ μέρη τοῦ σώματος κινοῦν καὶ δυνάμενον
ἐπί τε τὸ σφοδρότατον ἀνάγεσθαι καὶ ἐπὶ τὸ μαλα-
κώτατον ὑφίεσθαι τῶν μὲν ἄλλων οὐδέν, τοῦτο δὲ

equipment, as well as the freedom from em-
ployment to wait in leisure for the right occasion. However, the provision of the equipment
for the exercise with the small ball is accessible
even for the poorest, and the occasion of its enjoyment also awaits those who are very busy.
So, its accessibility is a very considerable benefit for its participants.

(5.902K) If you should consider each of the
exercises associated with the small ball—what
the exercise is capable of doing and what its nature is—you would especially understand that
it is the most comprehensive exercise. You will
find that it is vigorous or gentle, that it moves
the lower body parts more or the upper ones,
or that it moves some part rather than others
(for example, the muscles of the lower back, the
head, the hands, or the chest). No other exercise
is able to work all the parts of the body equally,
or to increase to a very vigorous pitch and abate

μόνον τὸ διὰ τῆς σμικρᾶς σφαίρας γυμνάσιον, ὀξύτα-
τόν <γ'> ἐν μέρει καὶ βραδύτατον γενόμενον, σφο-
δρότατόν τε καὶ πρᾳότατον, ὡς ἂν αὐτός τε βουληθῇς
καὶ τὸ σῶμα φαίνηται δεόμενον. οὕτω δὲ καὶ τὰ μέρη
κινεῖν ἔστι μὲν αὐτοῦ πάνθ' ὁμοῦ, εἰ τοῦτο συμφέρειν
δόξειεν, ἔστι δὲ πρὸ ἄλλων ἄλλα, εἰ καὶ τοῦτό ποτε
δόξειεν.

ὅταν μὲν γὰρ συνιστάμενοι πρὸς ἀλλήλους καὶ
ἀποκωλύοντες ὑφαρπάσαι τὸν μεταξὺ διαπονῶσι, μέ-
γιστον αὐτὸ καὶ σφοδρότατον καθίσταται πολλοῖς
μὲν τραχηλισμοῖς, πολλαῖς δ' ἀντιλήψεσι παλαιστικαῖς ἀναμεμιγμένον, ὥστε κεφαλὴν μὲν καὶ αὐχένα διαπονεῖσθαι τοῖς τραχηλισμοῖς, πλευρὰς δὲ
καὶ (5.903K) θώρακα καὶ γαστέρα ταῖς τε τῶν ἁμ-
μάτων περιθέσεσι καὶ ἀπώσεσι καὶ ἀποστηρίξεσι καὶ
ταῖς ἄλλαις παλαιστικαῖς λαβαῖς. τούτῳ δὲ καὶ ὀσφὺς
τείνεται σφοδρῶς καὶ σκέλη, <καὶ δὴ ῥώννυται καὶ
τὸ> ἑδραῖον τῆς βάσεως τῷ τοιούτῳ πόνῳ. τὸ δὲ καὶ

to a very gentle pitch: this is unique to the exercise with the small ball. The exercise may be very quick and very slow in turns, very vigorous or very mild, however you might wish it and however the body manifestly needs. And the exercise can move all parts of the body at the same time, if this should seem beneficial, or it can move some rather than others, if this too should ever seem preferable.

Whenever participants lined up across from one another work hard to keep each other from intercepting the ball, this is a very great and most vigorous exercise, which is combined with many neck grabs and many wrestling holds. As a result, the head and neck are exercised by the neck holds, while the lungs, **(5.903K)** chest, and abdomen are exercised by clinches, pushes, stances in position, and other wrestling holds. In this way too, the lower back and the legs are vigorously strained, and the firmness of one's

προβαίνειν <καὶ ὑποβαίνειν> καὶ εἰς τὰ πλάγια μεταπηδᾶν οὐ μικρὸν σκελῶν γυμνάσιον, ἀλλ', εἰ χρὴ τάληθὲς εἰπεῖν, μόνον δικαιότατα κινοῦν πάντ' αὐτῶν τὰ μόρια. τοῖς μὲν γὰρ προϊοῦσιν ἕτερα νεῦρα καὶ μύες, τοῖς δ' ὑποβαίνουσιν ἕτερα διαπονεῖται πλέον, οὕτω δὲ καὶ τοῖς εἰς τὰ πλάγια μεθισταμένοις ἄλλα. καὶ ὅστις καθ' ἓν εἶδος κινήσεως κινεῖ τὰ σκέλη καθάπερ οἱ θέοντες, ἀνωμάλως οὗτος καὶ ἀνίσως τὰ μέρη γυμνάζει.

(3) Ὡς δὴ τοῖς σκέλεσιν, οὕτω καὶ ταῖς χερσὶ τὸ γυμνάσιον τοῦτο δικαιότατον ἐν παντὶ σχήματι λαμβάνειν ἐθιζομένων τὴν σφαῖραν. ἀνάγκη γὰρ κἀνταῦθα τὴν ποικιλίαν τῶν σχημάτων ἄλλοτ' ἄλλους τῶν μυῶν τείνειν σφοδρότερον, ὥστε πάντας ἐν μέρει πονοῦντας ἴσον ἔχειν, (5.904K) ἀνάπαυλάν τε τοῖς ἡσυχάζουσιν εἶναι τὸν χρόνον τῶν ἐνεργούντων, καὶ

footing is also strengthened by such effort. Stepping forward and backward and lunging to each side are no light exercise for the legs, but to tell the truth, the only way to exercise all their parts in the most even way: for in stepping forward, some of the tendons and muscles are exercised, and in stepping backward others are exercised more, and similarly others in moving to the side. And whoever moves the legs in one type of movement, like runners do, exercises the parts unevenly and unequally.

(3) Indeed, just as for the legs, so also for the hands is this exercise the most balanced in every respect, since participants are accustomed to catch the ball. For necessarily here also, the variety of forms in which the exercise is undertaken strains some muscles quite vigorously at one time, and others at another time, so that all the muscles are worked equally in turn, **(5.904K)** and the time for those that are in action provides

οὕτως ἐν μέρει πάντας ἐνεργοῦντάς τε καὶ ἀναπαυο-
μένους οὔτ᾿ ἀργοὺς μένειν τὸ πάμπαν οὔτε κόποις
ἁλίσκεσθαι μόνους πονοῦντας. ὄψιν δ᾿ ὅτι γυμνάζει, μαθεῖν ἔνεστιν ὑπομνησθέντας, ὡς, εἰ μή τις
ἀκριβῶς τὴν ῥοπὴν τῆς σφαίρας εἰς ὅ τι φέροιτο προ-
αισθάνοιτο, διαμαρτάνειν τῆς λαβῆς ἀναγκαῖόν
ἐστιν αὐτόν.

ἐπὶ τούτῳ δὲ καὶ τὴν γνώμην θήγει τῇ φροντίδι
τοῦ τε μὴ καταβαλεῖν καὶ τοῦ διακωλῦσαι τὸν μέσον
ἢ αὐτὸν ὑφαρπάσαι, εἴ ἐν τούτῳ κατασταίη. φροντὶς
δὲ μόνη μὲν καταλεπτύνει, μιχθεῖσα δέ τινι γυμνα-
σίῳ καὶ φιλοτιμίᾳ καὶ εἰς ἡδονὴν τελευτήσασα τὰ μέγιστα καὶ τὸ σῶμα πρὸς ὑγίειαν καὶ τὴν ψυχὴν εἰς
σύνεσιν ὀνίνησιν. οὐ σμικρὸν δὲ καὶ τοῦτ᾿ ἀγαθόν,
ὅταν ἄμφω τὸ γυμνάσιον ὠφελεῖν δύνηται, καὶ σῶμα

a respite for those that are at rest. In this way, all muscles are in action and rest in turn, and no muscles remain completely idle nor do any succumb to exhaustion working alone. It is possible to understand that it exercises the vision, too, when one recalls that if a participant does not precisely predict the ball's momentum in the direction of its travel, he will necessarily miss the catch.

In addition to this, the exercise sharpens the mind because of the attention paid to not dropping the ball, or to blocking the player in the middle, or to oneself intercepting the ball, if he should be the one in the middle. Such mental preoccupation alone thins the body, but if mixed with some exercise and with ambitious rivalry, and if it also brings about pleasure, then it bestows the greatest benefits both on the body in terms of health and on the soul in terms of mental capacity. And this is no small good,

καὶ ψυχήν, εἰς τὴν ἰδίαν ἑκάτερον ἀρετήν. ὅτι δ᾽ ἀσκεῖν ἄμφω δύναται τὰς μεγίστας ἀσκήσεις, ἃς μάλιστα μετιέναι τοῖς στρατηγικοῖς οἱ πόλεως βασιλεῖς νόμοι κελεύουσιν. οὐ χαλεπὸν κατιδεῖν. ἐπιθέσθαι (5.905K) γὰρ ἐν καιρῷ καὶ λαθεῖν ἐπιθέμενον καὶ ὀξυλαβῆσαι τὴν πρᾶξιν καὶ σφετερίσασθαι τὰ τῶν ἐναντίων ἢ βιασάμενον ἢ καὶ ἀδοκήτως ἐπιθέμενον καὶ φυλάξαι τὰ κτηθέντα τῶν ἀγαθῶν στρατηγῶν ἔργα· καὶ τὸ σύμπαν φάναι, φύλακά τε καὶ φῶρα δεινὸν εἶναι χρὴ τὸν στρατηγόν, καὶ ταῦτ᾽ αὐτοῦ τῆς ὅλης τέχνης τὸ κεφάλαιον. ἆρ᾽ οὖν ἄλλο τι γυμνάσιον οὕτω προεθίζειν ἱκανὸν ἢ φυλάττειν τὸ κτηθὲν ἢ ἀνασῴζειν τὸ μεθειμένον ἢ τῶν ἐναντίων τὴν γνώμην προαισθάνεσθαι; θαυμάζοιμ᾽ ἄν, εἴ τις εἰπεῖν ἔχοι.

whenever an exercise is capable of benefitting both, that is the body and the soul, with a view to the excellence particular to each. It is not hard to see that the exercise with the small ball is able to provide both of the greatest forms of training, participation in which "the laws, rulers of the city" have enjoined on generals.[23] **(5.905K)** For the tasks of good generals are to attack at the right time, to attack with surprise, to seize the action swiftly, to appropriate the belongings of opponents (either by compelling them or by attacking them unexpectedly), and to guard what has been acquired—in sum, a general needs to be both a skilled guard and a thief, as these are the chief part of his entire craft. Is there any other exercise that so considerably trains someone to be accustomed beforehand to guard what has been acquired, to recover what has been lost, or to anticipate the intention of opponents? I would be surprised if anyone were able to say

τὰ πολλὰ γὰρ αὐτῶν αὐτὸ τοὐναντίον ἀργοὺς καὶ
ὑπνηλοὺς καὶ βραδεῖς τὴν γνώμην ἐργάζεται. καὶ γὰρ
καὶ ὅσα κατὰ παλαίστραν πονοῦσιν εἰς <πολλοὺς στε-
φανίτας ἀγῶνας,> πολυσαρκίαν μᾶλλον ἢ ἀρετῆς
ἄσκησιν φέρει· πολλοὶ γοῦν οὕτως ἐπαχύνθησαν, ὡς
δυσχερῶς ἀναπνεῖν. ἀγαθοί γ' οὐδ' ἂν <δύναινθ'> οἱ
τοιοῦτοι πολέμου γενέσθαι στρατηγοὶ ἢ βασιλικῶν ἢ
πολιτικῶν πραγμάτων ἐπίτροποι· θᾶττον ἂν τοῖς ὑσὶν
ἢ τούτοις τις ὁτιοῦν ἐπιτρέψειεν.

<ἀλλ'> ἴσως οἰήσῃ με δρόμον ἐπαινεῖν καὶ τἄλλ'
ὅσα λεπτύνει τὸ σῶμα γυμνάσια. τὸ δ' οὐχ **(5.906K)**
οὕτως ἔχει. τὴν γὰρ ἀμετρίαν ἐγὼ πανταχοῦ ψέγω,
καὶ πᾶσαν τέχνην ἀσκεῖν φημι χρῆναι τὸ σύμμετρον,
κἂν εἴ τι μέτρου στερεῖται, τοῦτ' οὐκ εἶναι καλόν.
οὔκουν οὐδὲ δρόμους ἐπαινῶ τῷ τε καταλεπτύνειν

so. Most exercises have the opposite effect and make men idle, drowsy, and slow in judgement. Indeed, however much athletes labor in the gym for a crown, all the more does this conduce to excessive bulkiness than to training in excellence. In fact, many men have been so fattened by this kind of training as to experience breathing difficulties. These kinds of men could not be generals who are good in war or be entrusted with the affairs of ruling or politics — one would more readily entrust anything to pigs than to men like these.[24]

But you will perhaps think that I am praising running and as many other exercises as thin the body. **(5.906K)** Not so: I object to imbalance everywhere and claim that every art needs to train good balance, and that if something lacks balance, it is not fine. Hence, I do not praise running since it has a tendency to thin the condition of the body and provides no training

τὴν ἕξιν καὶ τῷ μηδεμίαν ἄσκησιν ἀνδρείας ἔχειν. οὐ γὰρ δὴ τῶν ὠκέως φευγόντων τὸ νικᾶν, ἀλλὰ τῶν συστάδην κρατεῖν δυναμένων, οὐδὲ διὰ τοῦτο Λακεδαιμόνιοι πλεῖστον ἠδύναντο τῷ τάχιστα θεῖν, ἀλλὰ τῷ μένειν θαρροῦντες. εἰ δὲ καὶ πρὸς ὑγίειαν ἐξετάζοις, ἐφ᾽ ὅσον ἀνίσως γυμνάζει τὰ μέρη τοῦ σώματος, ἐπὶ τοσοῦτον οὐδ᾽ ὑγιεινόν. ἀνάγκη γὰρ αὐτῷ τὰ μὲν ὑπερπονεῖν, τὰ δ᾽ ἀργεῖν παντελῶς. οὐδέτερον δ᾽ αὐτῶν ἀγαθόν, ἀλλ᾽ ἄμφω καὶ νόσων ὑποτρέφει σπέρματα καὶ δύναμιν ἄρρωστον ἐργάζεται.

(4) Μάλιστ᾽ οὖν ἐπαινῶ γυμνάσιον, ὃ καὶ σώματος ὑγίειαν ἱκανὸν ἐκπορίζειν καὶ μερῶν εὐαρμοστίαν καὶ ψυχῆς ἀρετήν, ἃ πάντα τῷ διὰ τῆς σμικρᾶς σφαίρας ὑπάρχει. καὶ γὰρ ψυχὴν εἰς πάντα δυνατὸν (5.907K) ὠφελεῖν καὶ τοῦ σώματος τὰ μέρη δι᾽

for courage. Victory does not belong to those who flee swiftly, but to those who are able to prevail in hand-to-hand combat, and it was not because they were able to run very fast that the Spartans accomplished so much, but because they were courageous in standing firm. And if you should examine the matter too with a view to health, insofar as a person exercises the parts of his body unequally, to that extent, the exercise is unhealthy, since it is necessary that some parts be overworked while others remain completely idle. Neither of these is good, as both nourish the seeds of sickness and foster a weakened capacity.

(4) Therefore, I especially praise an exercise that provides considerably for health of the body along with concord of the parts and excellence of the soul, all of which are present in the exercise with the small ball. For in fact it is capable of (5.907K) helping the soul in every

ἴσου πάντα γυμνάζειν· ὃ καὶ μάλιστ᾽ εἰς ὑγίειαν συμ-
φέρει καὶ συμμετρίαν ἕξεως ἐργάζεται, μήτ᾽ ἄμετρον πολυσαρκίαν μήθ᾽ ὑπερβάλλουσαν ἰσχνότητα
φέρον, ἀλλ᾽ εἴς τε τὰς ἰσχύος δεομένας πράξεις ἱκανὸν
καὶ ὅσαι τάχους χρῄζουσιν ἐπιτήδειον. οὕτω μὲν οὖν
ὅσον ἐν αὐτῷ <τὸ> σφοδρότατον οὐδενὸς τῶν πάντων
κατ᾽ οὐδὲν ἀπολείπεται.

  τὸ δὲ πρᾳότατον ἴδωμεν αὖθις. ἔστι γὰρ ὅτε καὶ
τούτου δεόμεθα διά θ᾽ ἡλικίαν ἢ μηδέπω φέρειν ἰσχυ-
ροὺς πόνους ἢ μηκέτι δυνάμενοι καὶ κάματον ἐπα-
νεῖναι βουληθέντες ἢ ἐκ νόσων ἀνακομιζόμενοι. δοκεῖ
δέ μοι κἂν τούτῳ πλέον ἔχειν ἑτέρου παντός· οὐδὲν
γὰρ οὕτω πρᾷον <ὡς αὐτὸ τοῦτ᾽>, εἰ πρᾴως αὐτὸ με-
ταχειρίζοιο. δεῖ δὲ μέσῳ μὲν οὖν τηνικαῦτα χρῆσθαι

way and exercising all the parts of the body equally; and this is especially beneficial for health and brings about good balance in bodily state, without imbalanced fleshiness or excessive thinness, but is sufficient for activities requiring strength and suitable for as many activities as require speed. And so this exercise does not fall short of any other exercises, in any aspect, with respect to its vigorousness.

Let us look again at its great mildness. There are times when we need this, too, on account of age, either because we are not yet or no longer capable of handling strong physical exertion, or because we want to rest after painful physical labor, or because we are recovering from sickness. And it seems to me that the exercise with the small ball possesses this quality more than other exercises do, for no other activity is as mild as this one is, if you practice it mildly. This being the aim, a participant needs to take

μηδενὶ σύμμετρον ἀποστάντα, τὰ μὲν ἠρέμα προβαί-
νοντα, τὰ δὲ καὶ κατὰ χώραν μένοντα, μὴ πολλὰ
διαγωνισάμενον, ἐπὶ τῷδε <δὲ> τρίψεσι μαλακαῖς
δι' ἐλαίου καὶ λουτροῖς (5.908K) θερμοῖς χρῆσθαι.
τοῦτο μὲν <οὖν> ἀπάντων ἐστὶ πρᾳότατον, ὥστε καὶ
ἀναπαύσασθαι δεομένῳ συμφορώτατον εἶναι καὶ ἀρ-
ρώστου δύναμιν ἀνακαλέσασθαι δυνατώτατον καὶ
γέροντι καὶ παιδὶ συμφορώτατον.

ὅσα δὲ τούτου μὲν ἰσχυρότερα, τοῦ δ' ἄκρως σφο-
δροῦ πρᾳότερα διὰ τῆς σμικρᾶς σφαίρας ἐνεργεῖται,
χρὴ καὶ ταῦτα γιγνώσκειν, ὅστις γ' ὀρθῶς βούλεται
διὰ παντὸς αὐτὴν μεταχειρίζεσθαι. καὶ γὰρ εἴ ποτε
δι' ἀναγκαίων ἔργων, οἷά τινα πολλὰ πολλάκις ἡμᾶς
καταλαμβάνει, πονήσειας ἀμέτρως ἢ τοῖς ἄνω μέρεσι
καὶ τοῖς κάτω πᾶσιν ἢ ποσὶ μόνοις ἢ χερσίν, ἔνεστί
σοι διὰ τοῦδε τοῦ γυμνασίου τὰ μὲν ἀναπαῦσαι, τὰ

up a position in the middle and not deviate at all from good balance, sometimes stepping forward softly and sometimes remaining in place, not overly exerting himself, and afterward make use of gentle massages with olive oil and (5.908K) warm baths. This is, then, the mildest exercise of all, such that it is most beneficial for someone who needs to recover and most effective for restoring the capacity of someone who is weak. It is therefore most suitable for the elderly and for children.

Whoever rightly wishes to continually engage in the exercise with the small ball must also know about the stronger activities that can be done with it but which are milder than peak vigorousness. For if, during the required activities of the kind that are often imposed on us, you exert either the upper parts or all the lower ones in an imbalanced way, or the feet or hands alone, then you can, through this exercise, rest

πρότερον κεκμηκότα, τὰ δ' εἰς τὴν ἴσην ἐκείνοις κίνη-
σιν καταστῆσαι, τὰ πρότερον ἀργὰ παντελῶς μεμε-
νηκότα. τὸ μὲν γὰρ ἐκ διαστήματος ἱκανοῦ βάλλειν
εὐτόνως, ἢ οὐδὲν τοῖς σκέλεσιν ἢ παντάπασιν ὀλίγα
χρώμενον, ἀναπαύει μὲν τὰ κάτω, τὰ δ' ἄνω κινεῖ
σφοδρότερον· τὸ δ' ἐπὶ πλέον διαθέοντα καὶ ὠκέως
ἐκ πολλῶν διαστημάτων ὀλιγάκις προσχρῆσθαι τῇ
βολῇ τὰ κάτω μᾶλλον διαπονεῖ. καὶ τὸ μὲν ἠπειγμένον ἐν αὐτῷ (5.909K) καὶ ταχὺ χωρὶς συντονίας
ἰσχυρᾶς τὸ πνεῦμα μᾶλλον γυμνάζει· τὸ δ' εὔτονον
ἐν ταῖς ἀντιλήψεσι καὶ βολαῖς καὶ λαβαῖς, οὐ μὴν
ταχύ γε, τὸ σῶμα μᾶλλον ἐντείνει τε καὶ ῥώννυσιν· εἰ
δ' εὔτονόν θ' ἅμα καὶ ἠπειγμένον εἴη, διαπονήσει
τοῦτο μεγάλως καὶ τὸ σῶμα καὶ τὸ πνεῦμα καὶ πάντων ἔσται γυμνασίων σφοδρότατον.

ἐφ' ὅσον δὲ δεῖ καθ' ἑκάστην χρείαν ἐπιτείνειν
τε καὶ ἀνιέναι, γράψαι μὲν οὐχ οἷόν τε (τὸ γὰρ ἐν

the parts that were exhausted before and also bring into equal movement those parts that previously remained completely idle. Throwing intensely from a great distance involves the legs not at all, or very little, and allows one to rest the lower parts while moving the upper ones more vigorously. But if one runs more and more quickly and makes a throw from greater distances less often, then one exerts the lower parts more. And the urgency and speed in this, **(5.909K)** which is without strong strain, exercises the breath more, while the strenuous activity in the holds, throws, and catches, which are not quick, rather strains and strengthens the body. If the activity is both strenuous and urgent, then this will greatly exert both the body and the breath, and it will be the most vigorous of all exercises.

It is not possible to write down how much tension and relaxation of the muscles is needed

ἑκάστῳ ποσὸν ἄρρητον), ἐπ᾽ αὐτῶν δὲ τῶν ἔργων
εὑρεῖν τε καὶ διδάξαι δυνατόν, ἐν ᾧ δὴ καὶ μάλιστα
τὸ πᾶν κῦρος· οὐδὲ γὰρ ἡ ποιότης ἐστὶ χρήσιμος, εἰ
τῷ ποσῷ διαφθείροιτο. τοῦτο μὲν δὴ τῷ παιδοτρίβῃ
μεθείσθω τῷ μέλλοντι τὸ γυμνάσιον ὑφηγεῖσθαι.

(5) Τὸ δ᾽ ὑπόλοιπον τοῦ λόγου περαινέσθω. βούλο-
μαι γὰρ ἐφ᾽ οἷς εἶπον ἀγαθοῖς προσεῖναι τῷδε τῷ γυ-
μνασίῳ μηδ᾽ <οἵων τε καὶ> ὅσων ἐκτός ἐστι κινδύνων
παραλιπεῖν, οἷς τὰ πλεῖστα τῶν ἄλλων περιπίπτει.
δρόμοι μὲν γὰρ ὠκεῖς πολλοὺς ἤδη διέφθειραν, ἀγ-
γεῖον ἐπίκαιρον ῥήξαντες. οὕτω δὲ καὶ φωναὶ μεγάλαι
θ᾽ ἅμα καὶ σφοδραὶ καθ᾽ ἕνα χρόνον (5.910K) ἀθρόως
ἐκφωνηθεῖσαι μεγίστων κακῶν οὐκ ὀλίγοις αἴτιαι
<κατέστησαν. καὶ μέντοι> καὶ ἱππασίαι σύντονοι τῶν
τε κατὰ νεφροὺς ἔρρηξάν τι καὶ τῶν κατὰ θώρακα

in each case, because the degree in each particular case cannot be stated, but it is possible in
the course of the activities themselves to discover and teach these things, wherein lies the
whole value of the exercise. For the quality of
exercise is not useful if it is ruined by the degree.
This should be left in the hands of the physical
trainer who is going to instruct the exercise.

(5) Now to conclude the remainder of the
discussion. In adding to the good things I said
about this exercise, I do not want to overlook
what sort and how many dangers it is free of
that very often attend other exercises. Swift
running has already killed many after they rup-
ture a crucial blood vessel. Similarly, loud and
violent sounds all at once in the same moment
(5.910K) have been responsible for great ills
for not a few people. And furthermore, intense horse riding has broken some of the parts
around the kidneys and injured parts of the

πολλάκις ἔβλαψαν, ἔστι δ' ὅτε καὶ τοὺς σπερματι-
κοὺς πόρους, ἵνα τὰ τῶν ἵππων ἁμαρτήματα παρα-
λείπω, δι' ἅ γε πολλάκις ἐκπεσόντες τῆς ἕδρας οἱ
ἱππεῖς παραχρῆμα διεφθάρησαν. οὕτω δὲ καὶ τὸ ἅλμα
καὶ ὁ δίσκος καὶ τὰ διὰ τοῦ σκάπτειν γυμνάσια <πολ-
λοῖς μελῶν τι διέστρεψε γυμνασθεῖσιν.> τοὺς δ' ἐκ
τῆς παλαίστρας τί δεῖ καὶ λέγειν, ὡς ἅπαντες λελώ-
βηνται τῶν Ὁμηρικῶν Λιτῶν οὐδὲν μεῖον; ὡς γὰρ
ἐκείνας φησὶν ὁ ποιητὴς "χωλάς τε ῥυσάς τε παρα-
βλῶπάς τ' ὀφθαλμώ," οὕτω τοὺς ἐκ τῆς παλαίστρας
ἴδοις ἂν ἢ χωλοὺς ἢ διεστραμμένους ἢ τεθλασμένους
ἢ πάντως γέ τι μέρος πεπηρωμένους. εἰ δὴ πρὸς
οἷς εἶπον ἀγαθοῖς ἔτι καὶ τοῦθ' ὑπάρχει τοῖς διὰ
τῆς σμικρᾶς σφαίρας γυμνασίοις, ὡς μηδὲ κινδύνῳ
πελάζειν, ἁπάντων ἂν εἴη πρὸς ὠφέλειαν ἄριστα
παρεσκευασμένα.

chest, and sometimes also the spermatic ducts. This is to pass over errors made by the horses, because of which the riders, often falling off the back of the horse, are immediately killed. So also jumping exercises, the discus, and exercises related to digging have wrenched the limbs of many who are exercising. And do we even need to talk about those from the wrestling gyms by pointing out they are all mutilated no less than the prayers described by Homer? For just as the poet says that they are "lame, withered, and blind in the eyes,"[25] so you might see those come from the wrestling gyms: limping, crippled, disfigured, blind, or totally disabled in some body part. And if, besides all these good things I said, this too is true of the exercise with the small ball—that it is not dangerous— then surely it would provide the greatest benefit of all.

On Hygiene

This extensive treatise discusses hygiene—what we today might call wellness, or preventive care including diet and exercise—and dates to approximately 175 CE. Proper hygiene, Galen writes, ensures that the body remains in the well-mixed, balanced, healthy state that is unique to each individual. This section focuses on types of exercise, many of which can be done without any kind of equipment (and the others with only simple equipment, or with a training partner)—a practical feature that makes these activities useful indeed for ancient and modern readers alike!

Galen is particular in his use of vocabulary in order to characterize and to classify the nature of each exercise, an aspect of his writing that I have tried to preserve in translation through the careful use of words such as "vigorous," "forceful," "intense," and "powerful." We might find corollaries of his recognition that different types and intensities of physical exertion affect the body differently in the recommendations made by today's physicians and physical therapists: the condition of one's body and the presence of comorbidities affect the types and intensity of exercises that are recommended.

(6.139.9K) ἤδη δ᾽ ἐπὶ τὰ καθ᾽ ἕκαστον τῶν γυμνασίων ἴδια τὸν λόγον ἄγειν καιρός, ἐπισημηνάμενόν
γε πρότερον, ὡς καὶ κατὰ ταῦτα πλείους εἰσὶν αἱ διαφοραί. τὰ μὲν γὰρ ἄλλοτε ἄλλο τι μέρος ἕτερον
ἑτέρου γυμνάζει μᾶλλον, καὶ τὰ μὲν ἐλινυόντων γίνεται, τὰ δὲ ὀξύτατα κινουμένων, καὶ τὰ μὲν εὐτόνως,
τὰ δὲ ἀτόνως, καὶ πρὸς τούτοις ἔτι τὰ μὲν σφοδρῶς,
τὰ δ᾽ ἀμυδρῶς. εὔτονον μὲν οὖν γυμνάσιον ὀνο-
μάζω τὸ βιαίως ἄνευ τάχους διαπονοῦν, σφοδρὸν
δὲ τὸ βιαίως τε καὶ σὺν τάχει· βιαίως δὲ ἢ ῥω-
μαλέως (6.140K) λέγειν οὐ διοίσει.

τὸ μὲν οὖν σκάπτειν εὔτονόν τε καὶ ῥωμαλέον
ἐστίν, οὕτω δὲ καὶ τὸ τέτταρας ἵππους ἅμα κατέχειν
ἡνίαις εὔτονον μὲν ἱκανῶς γυμνάσιον, οὐ μὴν ὠκύ γε,

DIFFERENT TYPES OF EXERCISE

(6.139.9K) Now is the right occasion to have a discussion about the details of each of the exercises, first indicating that the differences among these are many: some exercise one part more than another (and at variable times); others are for recovery; others involve the quickest movements, others strenuous movements, others relaxed movements, and besides these, others that are done vigorously, and others that are done weakly. I term "intense" the exercise that works the body forcefully but without speed, and "vigorous" that which is done forcefully and with speed (**[6.140K]** but it will make no difference here whether we say "forcefully" or "powerfully").

So, digging is both intense and powerful, and holding back four horses at the same time with the reins is a considerably intense exercise, but

κατὰ δὲ τὸν αὐτὸν τρόπον, εἴ τις ἀράμενος ὁτιοῦν μέ-
γιστον φορτίον ἢ μένοι κατὰ χώραν ἢ προβαίνοι σμικρά. καὶ οἱ ἀνάντεις περίπατοι τούτου τοῦ γένους
εἰσίν· ἀναφέρεται γοῦν καὶ ἀναβαστάζεται κατ᾽
αὐτοὺς ὑπὸ τῶν πρώτων κινουμένων ὀργάνων ἅπαντα τὰ λοιπὰ μόρια τοῦ σώματος, ὥσπερ τι φορτίον.
οὕτω δὲ καὶ ὅστις ἀναρριχᾶται διὰ σχοινίου, καθάπερ
ἐν παλαίστρᾳ γυμνάζουσι τοὺς παῖδας εἰς εὐτονίαν παρασκευάζοντες. ὡσαύτως δὲ καὶ ὅστις ἢ
σχοινίου λαβόμενος ἤ τινος ὑψηλοῦ ξύλου μέχρι
πλείστου κατέχει κρεμάμενος ἐξ αὐτοῦ, ῥωμαλέον
μέν τι καὶ ἰσχυρὸν γυμνάζεται γυμνάσιον, οὐ μὴν
ὠκύ γε, καὶ ὅστις προτείνας ἢ ἀνατείνας τὼ χεῖρε
πὺξ ἔχων ἀτρεμίζει μέχρι πλείστου. εἰ δὲ καὶ πα-
ραστήσας τινὰ κελεύει καθέλκειν κάτω τὼ χεῖρε,
μὴ ἐνδιδοὺς αὐτός, ἔτι δὴ μᾶλλον οὗτος εἰς εὐρω-
στίαν παρασκευάζει τούς τε μῦς καὶ τὰ νεῦρα·

not a swift one and, similarly, if someone were to lift some very large burden and either stand in one place or walk a little. Walking uphill is also this kind of exercise; at any rate, the other parts of the body are lifted up and carried along by the primarily moving organs, as if they were some weight. And the same is true for someone climbing up a rope, as they train boys in the athletic gym, preparing them to be vigorous. In the same way, when someone, taking a rope or some high beam, holds on and hangs from it for as long as possible, he is performing a certain powerful and strong exercise, but not a quick one. The same is true for someone who keeps still for as long as possible while either stretching out or lifting up his hands with the fists clenched. And if he has someone stand next to him and tells him to press down on his hands, while holding his position, this trains his muscles and tendons to attain even greater power.

(6.141K) τούτων γὰρ ἴδια τὰ τοιαῦτα μάλιστα σύμπαντα γυμνάσια· πολὺ δὲ δὴ μᾶλλον, εἴ τι βάρος ταῖς χερσὶν ἄκραις περιλαβὼν ἑκατέραις καταμόνας, οἷοίπερ οἱ κατὰ παλαίστραν εἰσὶν ἁλτῆρες, ἀτρέμας ἔχει προτείνας ἢ ἀνατείνας αὐτάς. εἰ δὲ δὴ καὶ κελεύσειε τινι καθέλκειν τε καὶ κάμπτειν βιαίως, ἑαυτὸν ἀκίνητόν τε καὶ ἄκαμπτον οὐ ταῖς χερσὶ μόνον, ἀλλὰ καὶ τοῖς σκέλεσι καὶ τῇ ῥάχει διαφυλάττων, οὐ σμικρὸν γυμνάσεται γυμνάσιον εἰς εὐτονίαν ὀργάνων. οὕτω τοι λόγος ἔχει κἀκεῖνον τὸν Μίλωνα γυμνάζειν ἑαυτόν, ἐνίοτε μὲν ἀποσαλεῦσαί τε καὶ μετακινῆσαι τῆς ἕδρας ἐπιτρέποντα τῷ βουλομένῳ (ἀλλὰ τοῦτο μὲν σκελῶν ἂν εἴη μάλιστα γυμνάσιον), ἐνίοτε δέ, εἰ τὰς χεῖρας γυμνάζειν βούλοιτο, τὴν πυγμὴν διαλύειν κελεύοντα· αὖθις δ' <ἄν>, ὥς φασιν, ἐν ταῖν χεροῖν ἔχων ἢ ῥοιὰν ἢ ἕτερόν τι τοιοῦτον ἀφαιρεῖσθαι τῷ βουλομένῳ παρεῖχε.

(6.141K) All such exercises are especially specific to training the muscles and tendons, and they become even more so if someone, holding in each of his hands a weight like the kind the athletes in the wrestling school use, smoothly extends his arms out or up. Then, if he tells someone to try to pull his hands down, or to bend them forcefully, while he remains unmoved and rigid in not only his upper extremities, but also his legs and spine, he will be doing a significant exercise to strengthen his organs. So there is even a story that the famous Milo exercised similarly: he sometimes ordered anyone who wanted to attempt it to shake him loose and to remove him from his seat (this would be in particular a leg exercise), and sometimes, if he wished to exercise his hands, would tell someone to try to open his fists. Or, as the story goes, he would hold a pomegranate or other such

ταυτὶ μὲν οὖν τὰ γυμνάσια μεγίστης ἰσχύος ἐπί-
δειξίν τε ἅμα καὶ ἄσκησιν ἔχει, τόνον δὲ μορίων
γυμνάζει τε καὶ ῥώννυσι, (6.142K) κἀπειδὰν ἤτοι
διαλαβὼν ἕτερόν τινα μέσον ἢ διαληφθεὶς αὐτὸς
ἐπηλλαγμένων πρὸς ἀλλήλας τῶν χειρῶν τε καὶ τῶν
δακτύλων ἤτοι τῷ κρατουμένῳ προστάξῃ διαλύειν ἢ
αὐτὸς λύῃ τοῦ κρατοῦντος· οὕτω δὲ κἀπειδάν, ἑτέρου
προνεύσαντος ἐκ πλαγίων αὐτῷ προσελθὼν ἐν κύκλῳ
τοῖς λαγόσι περιβαλὼν τὰς χεῖρας, ὥσπερ γέ τι φορτίον ἀράμενος ἀναφέρῃ τε ἅμα καὶ περιφέρῃ τὸν
ἀρθέντα, καὶ μᾶλλον εἰ ἐπινεύοι τε καὶ ἀνανεύοι βα-
στάζων· ὧδε γὰρ ἂν ἀκριβῶς τις ἅπασαν τὴν ῥάχιν
εἰς ῥώμην παρασκευάσειεν. οὕτω δὲ καὶ ὅσοι τὰ
στέρνα πρὸς ἀλλήλους ἀπερεισάμενοι βιαίως ὠθοῦσιν

thing in his hands, and he would present it to whoever wanted to try to take it.

These exercises are at the same time a display of the greatest strength and also are training, and they exercise the tension of the parts and empower them: **(6.142K)** for example, whenever someone, grabbing hold of another wrestler around the middle—or whenever he himself is held this way—overlaps his hands and fingers with each other in his grip, and then bids the one holding him to release him, or frees himself from the one holding on to him; likewise, whenever someone approaches a bent-over opponent from the side and wraps his hands around his opponent's middle along his flanks, and lifting him up like a burden, simultaneously carries him around held high, and even more so if he bends forward and backward while holding him. In this manner someone could, in a precise way, train his whole spine to become powerful.

εἰς τοὐπίσω καὶ ὅσοι τῶν αὐχένων ἐκκρεμάμενοι κατασπῶσιν, εἰς εὐτονίαν παρασκευάζουσιν.

ἀλλὰ τὰ μὲν τοιαῦτα καὶ χωρὶς παλαίστρας ἢ βαθείας κόνεως δύναται γίνεσθαι καθ' ὁτιοῦν χωρίον ἐπίκροτον ὀρθῶν ἑστώτων· ὅσα δὲ παλαίοντες εἰς ἀλλήλους δρῶσιν ἀσκοῦντες τὸν τόνον, ἤτοι κόνεως βαθείας ἢ παλαίστρας δεῖται. ἔστι δὲ τὰ τοιάδε· περιπλέξαντες τοῖς ἑαυτοῦ δύο σκέλεσι τὸ ἕτερον σκέλος τοῦ προσπαλαίοντος, ἔπειθ' ἅψαντες πρὸς ἀλλήλας τὼ χεῖρε, (6.143K) τὴν μὲν ἐπὶ τὸν αὐχένα βιαίως ἐρείδειν, ἥτις ἂν ᾖ κατ' εὐθὺ τοῦ κατειλημμένου σκέλους, τὴν δ' ἑτέραν ἐπὶ τὸν βραχίονα. δύναιτο δ' ἂν καὶ περὶ τὴν κεφαλὴν ἄκραν τὸ ἅμμα περιθεὶς ἀνακλᾶν εἰς τοὐπίσω βιαζόμενος. τὰ τοιαῦτα γὰρ παλαίσματα πρὸς εὐτονίαν ἑκάτερον τῶν παλαιόντων ἀσκεῖ, καθάπερ γε καὶ ὅσα ζώσαντος τοῖς σκέλεσι θατέρου τὸ ἕτερον ἢ κατ' ἀμφοῖν ἄμφω

Similarly, those who bring their chests together and forcefully push against each other and those who pull downward when hanging from their necks are training to be vigorous.[26]

But it is also possible to do such exercises outside the athletic gym or the deep sand, while standing in place on well-packed ground; all the exercises the wrestlers do with one another while strength training need deep sand or the athletic gym, however. These include when a wrestler folds both his own legs around the leg of his opponent **(6.143K)** and then forcefully leans on the neck with his hands interlaced, with one hand on the same side as the leg in the hold, and the other hand on the opponent's arm. And he might also place his clinch hold around the top of his opponent's head and forcibly bend it backward. Such strenuous maneuvers train each one of the wrestlers to be powerful, just when one has wrapped his two legs around the

καθέντος γίνεται· καὶ γὰρ καὶ ταῦτ' ἀμφότερα εἰς ῥώμην παρασκευάζει.

μυρία δὲ ἕτερα τοιαῦτα κατὰ παλαίστραν ἐστὶν εὔτονα γυμνάσια, περὶ ὧν ἁπάντων τὴν ἐμπειρίαν τε ἅμα καὶ τριβὴν ὁ παιδοτρίβης ἔχει, ἕτερος δέ τις ὢν ὅδε τοῦ γυμναστοῦ, καθάπερ ὁ μάγειρος τοῦ ἰατροῦ. καί πως ἔοικεν αὖ καὶ τοῦθ' ἡμῖν ἥκειν εἰς σκέμμα· περὶ οὗ λέλεκται μὲν ἤδη καὶ κατ' ἐκεῖνο τὸ βιβλίον, ὃ Θρασύβουλον ἐπιγράφομεν, εἰρήσεται δὲ καὶ νῦν ὅσον αὔταρκες εἰς τὰ παρόντα, πρότερόν γε διελθόντων ἡμῶν τὰς τῶν γυμνασίων διαφοράς. ὅσα μὲν οὖν εὔτονα, καὶ δὴ λέλεκται.

(6.144K) Μεταβαίνειν δὲ ἤδη καιρὸς ἐπὶ τὰ ταχέα χωρὶς εὐτονίας καὶ βίας. δρόμοι δ' εἰσὶ ταῦτα καὶ σκιομαχίαι καὶ ἀκροχειρισμοὶ καὶ τὸ διὰ τοῦ κωρύκου τε καὶ τῆς σμικρᾶς σφαίρας γυμνάσιον, ὅταν ἐκ διεστώτων τε καὶ διαθεόντων γίνηται. τοιοῦτον δέ τι καὶ τὸ ἐκπλεθρίζειν ἐστὶ καὶ τὸ πιτυλίζειν. τὸ μὲν

other's leg or around both: both maneuvers foster the development of power.

There are innumerable other such intense exercises in the athletic gym, and the physical trainer is experienced and practiced in all of them, but he is as different from the athletic trainer as the cook is from the physician. (It seems that I have already examined this issue and discussed it previously in a book I entitled *Thrasybulus*.)[27] As many things as are sufficient for the current topic will now be discussed, first going through the differences between the gymnastic exercises. The intense ones have already been described.

(6.144K) Now it is the right occasion to pass on to the exercises that are fast, but not intense and forceful.[28] Running, shadow boxing, arm wrestling, the exercise with the punching bag, and the exercise with the small ball are these kinds, whether they happen while standing at a

ἐκπλεθρίζειν ἐστίν, ἐπειδάν τις ἐν πλέθρῳ πρόσω τε
ἅμα καὶ ὀπίσω διαθέων ἐν μέρει πολλάκις ἐφ' ἑκάτερα
χωρὶς καμπῆς ἀφαιρῇ τοῦ μήκους ἑκάστοτε βραχὺ
καὶ τελευτῶν εἰς ἓν καταστῇ βῆμα· τὸ δὲ πιτυλίζειν,
ἐπειδὰν ἐπ' ἄκρων τῶν ποδῶν βεβηκὼς ἀνατείνας
τὼ χεῖρε κινῇ τάχιστα, τὴν μὲν ὀπίσω φέρων, τὴν δὲ
πρόσω. μάλιστα δὲ τοίχῳ προσιστάμενοι γυμνάζο-
νται τοῦτο τὸ γυμνάσιον, ἵν', εἰ καί ποτε σφάλλοι-
ντο, προσαψάμενοι τοῦ τοίχου ῥᾳδίως ὀρθῶνται· καὶ
οὕτω δὴ γυμναζομένων λανθάνει τε τὰ σφάλματα καὶ
ἀσφαλέστερον γίνεται τὸ γυμνάσιον. ὠκεῖαι δὲ κινήσεις εἰσίν, οὐ μὴν βίαιοί γε, καὶ ὅσαι κατὰ παλαίστραν ἐπιτελοῦνται κυλινδουμένων ὀξέως (6.145K)
μεθ' ἑτέρων τε καὶ καταμόνας. ἐγχωρεῖ δὲ καὶ ὀρθοὺς

distance or while running. Interval running and weighted arm swings, too, are in this category. Interval running is whenever someone, running forward and then back for a distance of one hundred feet multiple times, without turning to either side, decreases the distance a little with each interval until he stops at one step. And weighted arm swings are when someone, balancing on tiptoe, extends his arms and moves them very fast, driving them backward and forward. Most often, people doing this exercise stand against a wall, so that, if they stumble at some point, they can easily right themselves by grabbing the wall. But for those exercising in this way, their stumbles escape their notice, and the exercise becomes less effective. Furthermore, those movements are quick, but not forceful, however many are done in the gym as people tumble quickly, **(6.145K)** either with others or individually. It is also possible to do a

ἐνειλουμένους τε ἅμα καὶ μεταβαλόντας ἐν τάχει τὸν
πέλας ὀξὺ γυμνάσασθαι γυμνάσιον. ἐγχωρεῖ δὲ καὶ
διὰ τῶν σκελῶν μόνων ὀρθὸν ἐφ' ἑνὸς χωρίου γυμνάσασθαι γυμνάσιον ὀξύ, πολλάκις μὲν εἰς τοὐπίσω
μόνον ἐφαλλόμενον, ἔστιν ὅτε δὲ καὶ εἰς τοὔμπροσθεν
ἀναφέροντα τῶν σκελῶν ἑκάτερον ἐν μέρει. καὶ μὲν
δὴ καὶ διὰ τῶν χειρῶν ἔστιν ὀξὺ γυμνάσιον ὁμοιόρρο-
πον γυμνάσασθαι χωρὶς τοῦ κατέχειν ἁλτῆρας, ἐπι-
σπεύδοντα τὰς κινήσεις αὐτῶν εἰς πυκνότητά τε
ἅμα καὶ τάχος, εἴτε πὺξ ἐθέλοι τις εἴτε καὶ χωρὶς πυγ-
μῆς ἀνασείειν ἁπλῶς. τοιοῦτον μὲν δή τι καὶ τὸ ταχὺ
γυμνάσιόν ἐστιν ἐν οἷς εἴπομεν εἴδεσιν ἀφωρισμένον.

ἐπὶ δὲ τὸ σφοδρὸν ἰέναι καιρός. ἔστι δ', ὡς εἴρηται, τοῦτο σύνθετον ἐξ εὐτόνου τε καὶ ταχέος. ὅσα
γὰρ εὔτονα τῶν γυμνασίων εἴρηται, τούτοις ἅπασιν
ὡς σφοδροῖς ἄν τις χρῶτο, ταχείας κινήσεις προστι-
θείς. οὐχ ἥκιστα δὲ καὶ τὰ τοιάδε γυμνάσια σφοδρά,

quick exercise by standing upright and engaging with, and at the same time changing positions with, the person nearest with speed. It is also often possible to do a quick exercise with the legs alone standing upright in one place, by frequently lunging backward only and then again lunging each leg forward in turns. And it is also possible to exercise the hands quickly in a similar way without holding on to the weights, by accelerating the frequency and speed of the movements at the same time, either with the hands in fists, or simply swinging the hands to and fro without making fists. Of such a sort is the [category of] fast exercise, divided into the into types I mentioned.

Now we will discuss vigorous exercise. It is, as I said, a composite of intense and fast exercise. Someone might use as strenuous exercise all those exercises described as vigorous, with the addition of fast movements. And these

σκάψαι καὶ δισκεῦσαι [καὶ κινῆσαι] καὶ πηδῆσαι συνεχῶς ἄνευ τοῦ διαναπαύεσθαι. (6.146K) οὕτω δὲ
καὶ τὸ ἀκοντίζειν ὁτιοῦν τῶν βαρέων βελῶν συνείρο-
ντα τὴν ἐνέργειαν ἢ βαρέσιν ὅπλοις ἐσκεπασμένον
ἐνεργεῖν ὀξέως. ἀμέλει καὶ οἱ γυμναζόμενοι διά τινος
τῶν τοιούτων ἀναπαύονται κατὰ βραχύ. καί σοι καὶ
ἡ κατὰ τὸ συνεχές τε καὶ διαλεῖπον γυμνάσιον ἤδη
πως γινωσκέσθω διαφορά. τὰ γὰρ εἰρημένα νῦν δὴ
πάντα διαλείποντες μᾶλλον εἰς χρείαν ἄγουσι, καὶ
μάλισθ᾽ ὅσα πόνοι τινές εἰσι καὶ ἔργα, μὴ μόνον γυμνάσια, καθάπερ τὸ ἐρέσσειν τε καὶ σκάπτειν. ὅσα δ᾽
ἀσθενέστερα τῶν γυμνασίων ἐστίν, ἄνευ τοῦ διαναπαύεσθαι γίνεται μᾶλλον, ὥσπερ ὁ δόλιχός τε καὶ αἱ
ὁδοιπορίαι.

Ταῦτ᾽ οὖν ἄπαντα γυμνασίων ἐστὶν εἴδη, τάς γε
νῦν εἰρημένας ἔχοντα διαφοράς καὶ πρὸς τούτοις ἔτι
τὸ τὰ μὲν ὀσφὺν μᾶλλον ἢ χεῖρας ἢ σκέλη διαπονεῖν,

exercises are also not least vigorous: digging, throwing rings around a peg, and jumping continuously without resting at intervals. **(6.146K)** Similarly, throwing any heavy weapons without interruption in the activity or acting quickly while wearing heavy armor are also intense exercises. To be sure, those who do one of these kinds of exercises stop after a little while. (And you should understand this as the distinction between continuous and interval exercise.) All these exercises presently under discussion are more interval exercises, especially those that are hard labor and work (and not only exercises), like rowing and digging. All weaker exercises more often occur without an interval, like distance running and walking.

So these are all the kinds of exercises, with their differences described, and besides these, there are those that exercise the low back, the hands, or the legs more, or the whole spine,

τὰ δὲ τὴν ῥάχιν ὅλην ἢ τὸν θώρακα μόνον ἢ τὸν πνεύμονα. βάδισις μέν γε καὶ δρόμος ἴδια σκελῶν γυμνάσια, ἀκροχειρισμοὶ δὲ καὶ σκιομαχίαι ἴδια χειρῶν, ὀσφύος δὲ τὸ ἐπικύπτειν τε καὶ ἀνακύπτειν συνεχῶς **(6.147K)** ἢ αἴροντά τι βάρος ἀπὸ τῆς γῆς ἢ ἐν ταῖν χειροῖν βαστάζοντά τι διαπαντός. ἔνιοι μὲν γὰρ καταθέντες ἅλτῆρας ἐν τῷ πρόσθεν διεστῶτας ἀλλήλων ὀργυιάν, εἶτ' ἐν τῷ μέσῳ στάντες αὐτῶν ἀναιροῦνται προκύπτοντες, τῇ μὲν δεξιᾷ χειρὶ τὸν ἐν τοῖς ἀριστεροῖς, τῇ δὲ ἀριστερᾷ τὸν ἐν τοῖς δεξιοῖς, καὶ αὖθις ἑκάτερον εἰς τὴν οἰκείαν κατατίθενται χώραν καὶ τοῦτο δρῶσιν ἐφεξῆς πολλάκις ἀτρεμίζοντες τῇ βάσει. τὰ δὲ πλάγια μέρη τῆς ῥάχεως ἡ κίνησις ἥδε διαπονεῖ μᾶλλον, ὥσπερ ἡ προειρημένη τὰ κατ' εὐθύ.

or the chest alone, or the lungs. Walking and running are exercises particularly for the legs, wrestling and shadow boxing particularly for the upper extremities, and successively bending forward or backward **(6.147K)** or lifting some weight from the ground or gradually raising something in both hands continuously are particularly for the low back. Some people, putting weights down in front of them separated from each other by six feet, then stand in between them and bend forward and downward to lift up the weights, the one on the left in the right hand, and the one on the right in the left hand. They then place each back in its original location, doing this repeatedly while remaining still in a fixed position. This movement especially works the side parts of the spine, just as the aforementioned exercise works the central part of the spine.

3

Individual Physiologies

Perhaps one of the most remarkable aspects of Galen's approach to medicine involves his emphasis on the uniqueness of each individual. Every person had his or her own baseline internal mixture, influenced by parentage, environment, diet, activity, age, and a host of other factors. A skilled physician could characterize this internal mixture through touch and observation and could, by these same mechanisms, also identify derangements and provide individualized therapies to correct them. The importance of attaining the proper mixture and balance among hot, cold, wet, and dry — which was unique to each particular patient — was one of the foundations of Galen's theoretical and

practical approaches to medicine. He discusses these concepts in multiple texts, both those that mention this theory explicitly, and those that rely on it implicitly as an assumption in the diagnosis, prognosis, and treatment of disease.

Mixtures 1.5 and 2.4

This three-part text outlines Galen's view of humoral balance, how to determine a patient's unique internal balance, and what happens in cases of various bad mixtures. Earlier scientific theories, articulated by Aristotle, among others, had outlined four fundamental qualities: hot, cold, wet, and dry. The primary elements (those things are the indivisible components of the natural world and compose all other substances) of earth, air, water, and fire are associated with each of these qualities. The four bodily fluids (phlegm, black bile, yellow bile, blood) are characterized by combinations of the four funda-

mental qualities: phlegm was cold and wet, black bile was cold and dry, yellow bile was hot and dry, and blood was hot and wet.[29] *"Mixtures" is often read alongside Galen's other texts that describe humoral mixtures, symptoms, conditions, and diseases, and Galen himself considered it prerequisite reading for students prior to their engagement with his more extensive and comprehensive texts. Since this is one of Galen's more theoretical texts, it can be challenging to read. I have included it because Galen's clear insistence on health as a spectrum, defined by functionality, is remarkably modern. For example, Galen explicitly articulates a conception of "What is normal for you?"—that is, for an individual patient, in light of that person's characteristics and lifestyle—a perspective that characterizes current patient-centered approaches to diagnosis and treatment. As Galen writes in one of the included texts, "it is necessary to assume a wide*

(1.544.16K) Ἐπεὶ δὲ πολλὰ τὰ γένη, καθάπερ οὖν καὶ τὰ ἄτομα, δυνήσεται ταὐτὸν σῶμα καὶ θερμὸν καὶ ψυχρὸν καὶ ξηρὸνκαὶ ὑγρὸν εἶναι (1.545K) κατὰ πολλοὺς τρόπους. ἀλλ' ὅταν μὲν ἑνὶ τῷ τυχόντι παραβάλληται, πάνυ σαφές ἐστιν, ὡς ἐγχωρεῖ τἀναντία λέγεσθαι ταὐτόν, οἷον Δίωνα Θέωνος μὲν καὶ Μέμνονος ξηρότερον, Ἀρίστωνος δὲ καὶ Γλαύκωνος ὑγρότερον. ὅταν δὲ πρὸς τὸ σύμμετρον ὁμογενὲς ἢ ὁμοειδές, ἐνταῦθ' ἤδη συγχεῖσθαί τε καὶ ταράττεσθαι συμβαίνει τοὺς ἀγυμνάστους.

latitude for the healthy state." Yet at the same time, Galen (also like a modern physician) recognizes that there is an ideal disease-free state of perfect functionality, and that it is desirable for patients to reach this state.

PRECISION MEDICINE, OF A SORT

(1.544.16K) Since there are many genera and so also many individuals, it will be possible for the same body to be hot, cold, dry, and wet **(1.545K)** in many ways. But whenever a comparison is made in one random instance, it is abundantly clear that it is possible for opposites to be counted as the same, saying, for example, that Dion is drier than Theon and Memnon, and wetter than Ariston and Glaucon.[30] But whenever it regards good balance within the same genus or species, then it immediately turns out that those who are untrained are thrown into confusion and disorder. For the same man can

ὁ γὰρ αὐτὸς ἄνθρωπος ὑγρὸς ἅμα καὶ θερμὸς εἶναι δύναται καὶ ξηρὸς καὶ ψυχρός, ξηρὸς μὲν καὶ ψυχρὸς ὡς πρὸς τὸν σύμμετρον ἄνθρωπον παραβαλλόμενος, ὑγρὸς δὲ καὶ θερμὸς ὡς πρὸς ἄλλο τι ἢ ζῷον ἢ φυτὸν ἢ οὐσίαν ἡντινοῦν, οἷον ὡς πρὸς μὲν ζῷον, εἰ τύχοι, μέλιττάν τε καὶ μύρμηκα, πρὸς δὲ φυτὸν ἐλαίαν ἢ συκῆν ἢ δάφνην, πρὸς οὐσίαν δέ τιν' ἑτέραν, ἢ μήτε ζῷόν ἐστι μήτε φυτόν, οἷον λίθον ἢ σίδηρον ἢ χαλκόν. ἐν τούτοις δὲ τὸ μὲν πρὸς ἄνθρωπον παραβάλλειν πρὸς ὁμοειδές ἐστι παραβάλλειν, τὸ δὲ πρὸς μέλιτταν ἢ μύρμηκα πρὸς ὁμογενές, ὡσαύτως δὲ καὶ πρὸς φυτὸν ὁτιοῦν. ἔστι γὰρ **(1.546K)** ἀνωτέρω τοῦ ζῴου τοῦτο τὸ γένος, ὥσπερ οὖν καὶ αὐτοῦ τούτου λίθος καὶ σίδηρος καὶ χαλκὸς ἐκ τῶν ἄνωθεν γενῶν.

καλείσθω γοῦν <πρὸς> ὁμογενὲς ἕνεκα συντόμου διδασκαλίας ἡ τοιαύτη σύμπασα παραβολή, τοσόνδε

at the same time be both wet and hot and also dry and cold in comparison to a man who is well balanced, and wet and hot in comparison with some other thing such as an animal, a plant, or any other substance. For example, comparison may be made in relation to an animal, to the bee or ant perhaps; in relation to a plant, to the fig, laurel, or bay; and in relation to some other substance that is neither animal nor plant, to some such as stone, iron, or bronze. To compare, among these things, a man to another man is comparison within the same species, while comparing a man to a bee or ant is comparison within the same genus, as it also is to make a comparison with any plant, **(1.546K)** since this genus is higher than that of animal, just as stone, iron, and bronze belong to genera above that.[31]

For the sake of concise instruction, let every such comparison be called a comparison within

μόνον ἐν αὐτῇ διελομένων ἡμῶν, ὡς, ἐπειδὰν μὲν
ἁπλῶς οὐσία τις εὔκρατος λέγηται καὶ ταύτης δέ τις
ἑτέρα ξηροτέρα καὶ θερμοτέρα καὶ ψυχροτέρα καὶ
ὑγροτέρα, τὴν μὲν εὔκρατον ἐνταῦθα τὴν ἐκ τῶν ἐναντίων ἀκριβῶς ἴσων συνελθόντων ὀνομάζομεν, ὅσον
δ' ἀπολείπεται τῆσδε καὶ πλεονεκτεῖ κατά τι, τῷ τοῦ
πλεονεκτοῦντος ὀνόματι προσαγορεύομεν· ἐπειδὰν δ'
ἤτοι φυτὸν εὔκρατον ἢ ζῷον ὁτιοῦν εἴπωμεν, οὐκέθ'
ἁπλῶς ἀλλήλοις ἐν τῇ τοιαύτῃ λέξει τἀναντία παρα-
βάλλομεν, ἀλλὰ πρὸς τὴν τοῦ φυτοῦ φύσιν ἢ τὴν τοῦ
ζῴου τὴν ἀναφορὰν ποιούμεθα, συκῆν μὲν εὔκρατον,
εἰ τύχοι, λέγοντες, ὅταν, οἷα μάλιστα πρέπει τὴν
φύσιν ὑπάρχειν συκῇ, τοιαύτη τις ᾖ, κύνα δ' αὖ
καὶ σῦν καὶ ἵππον καὶ ἄνθρωπον, ἐπειδὰν καὶ τούτων ἕκαστον (1.547K) ἄριστα τῆς οἰκείας ἔχῃ φύσεως. αὐτὸ δὲ δὴ τοῦτο τὸ τῆς οἰκείας φύσεως ἔχειν

the same genus, making an exception here only to the extent that whenever some substance is called absolutely well mixed, and some other substance is drier, hotter, colder, or wetter, then we call that substance well mixed that is made up of opposites coming together precisely equally, and that to the extent that a substance falls short of or exceeds this well-mixed substance in some respect, we call it by the name of whatever is in excess. Whenever we speak of any well-mixed plant or animal, however, we no longer simply compare opposites to one another in this kind of utterance, but we make reference to the nature of the plant or of the animal, speaking of a well-mixed fig tree, for example, whenever it is of some such sort as the fig tree is most fittingly in its nature, and again of a well-mixed dog, pig, horse, or human, whenever each **(1.547K)** is in the best state with regard to its own nature. For something to be best

ἄριστα ταῖς ἐνεργείαις κρίνεται. καὶ γὰρ καὶ φυτὸν καὶ ζῷον ὁτιοῦν ἄριστα διακεῖσθαι τηνικαῦτά φαμεν, ὅταν ἐνεργήσῃ κάλλιστα. συκῆς μὲν γὰρ ἀρετὴ βέλτιστά τε καὶ πλεῖστα τελεσφορεῖν σῦκα· κατὰ ταὐτὰ δὲ καὶ τῆς ἀμπέλου τὸ πλείστας τε καὶ καλλίστας ἐκφέρειν σταφυλάς, ἵππου δὲ τὸ θεῖν ὠκύτατα καὶ κυνὸς εἰς μὲν θήρας τε καὶ φυλακὰς ἄκρως εἶναι θυμοειδῆ, πρὸς δὲ τοὺς οἰκείους πρᾳότατον.

  Ἅπαντ᾽ οὖν ταῦτα, τά τε ζῷα λέγω καὶ τὰ φυτά, τὴν ἀρίστην τε καὶ μέσην ἐν τῷ σφετέρῳ γένει κρᾶσιν ἔχειν ἐροῦμεν οὐχ ἁπλῶς, ὅταν ἰσότης ἀκριβὴς ᾖ τῶν ἐναντίων, ἀλλ᾽ ὅταν ἡ κατὰ δύναμιν αὐτοῖς ὑπάρχῃ συμμετρία. τοιοῦτον δέ τι καὶ τὴν δικαιοσύνην εἶναί φαμεν, οὐ σταθμῷ καὶ μέτρῳ τὸ ἴσον, ἀλλὰ τῷ προσήκοντί γε καὶ κατ᾽ ἀξίαν ἐξετάζουσαν. ἰσότης οὖν κράσεως ἐν ἅπασι τοῖς εὐκράτοις ζῴοις τε καὶ φυτοῖς ἐστιν, οὐχ ἡ κατὰ τὸν τῶν κερασθέντων

with regard to its own nature is judged by its functions. For in fact we say that any plant or animal is in the best condition at that time, whenever it carries out its functions in the best way. The excellence for a fig tree involves producing the best and most figs. In the same way, the excellence for a vine involves producing the most and finest grapes; for a horse, running the fastest; and for a dog, being the fiercest in hunting and guarding, but gentlest toward those in its household.

We will say that all these things, I mean both the plants and the animals, have the best and mean mixture within their own genus not simply whenever there is a precise equality of opposites, but in accordance with their capacity. We also say that justice is something like this, assessing equality not by weight and measure, but according to what is appropriate and fitting. Therefore, the equality of mixture in all well-mixed animals

στοιχείων ὄγκον, ἀλλ᾽ (1.548K) ἢ τῇ φύσει τοῦ τε ζῴου καὶ τοῦ φυτοῦ πρέπουσα. πρέπει δ᾽ ἔσθ᾽ ὅτε τὸ μὲν ὑγρὸν τοῦ ξηροῦ, τὸ δὲ ψυχρὸν τοῦ θερμοῦ πλέον ὑπάρχειν. οὐ γὰρ ὁμοίαν χρὴ κρᾶσιν ἔχειν ἄνθρωπον καὶ λέοντα καὶ μέλιτταν καὶ κύνα.

(1.609K) ἐπιδέδεικται γὰρ ἡμῖν καὶ δι᾽ ἄλλων, ὡς ἀναγκαῖόν ἐστιν οὐ σμικρὸν ὑποθέσθαι πλάτος τῆς ὑγιεινῆς καταστάσεως· ἀλλὰ καὶ νῦν φαίνεται σχεδὸν ἐν ὅλῳ τῷ λόγῳ τὴν μὲν εὔκρατόν τε καὶ μέσην φύσιν οἷον κανόνα τινὰ τῶν ἄλλων ἀεὶ τιθεμένων ἡμῶν, ὅσαι δ᾽ ἐφ᾽ ἑκάτερα τῆσδε, δυσκράτους ἀποφαινόντων· ὅπερ οὐκ ἂν ἦν, εἰ μὴ τὸ μᾶλλόν τε καὶ ἧττον ἡ ὑγιεινὴ κατάστασις ἐδέχετο. ἄλλη μὲν γὰρ ἐστιν ἡ ὑγιεινή, ἄλλη δ᾽ ἡ νοσώδης δυσκρασία· νοσώδης μὲν ἡ ἐπὶ πλεῖστον ἀποκεχωρηκυῖα τῆς εὐκράτου, ὑγιεινὴ δ᾽ ἡ ἐπ᾽ ὀλίγον. ὁρίσαι δ᾽ οὐδ᾽ ἐνταῦθα μέτρῳ καὶ σταθμῷ τὸ ποσὸν ἐγχωρεῖ, ἀλλ᾽ ἱκανὸν

and plants is not according to the mass of their mixed elements, but **(1.548K)** according to the equality that is fitting for the nature of the animal or the plant. It is appropriate that sometimes the wet exceed the dry, or the cold exceed the hot, since a man, a lion, a bee, and a dog need not have the same mixture. . . .

(1.609.1K) For it was shown by us elsewhere that it is necessary to assume a wide latitude for the healthy state. It also clear now in practically our entire argument, however, since we continually set down the well-mixed and mean nature as a sort of standard for the rest and show that as many natures are outside of this range are badly mixed. This would not be the case unless the healthy state admitted greater and lesser degrees. Hence, the healthy bad mixture is one kind, and the sick bad mixture another: the sick badly mixed state departs most from the well

γνώρισμα τῆς ὑγιεινῆς δυσκρασίας τὸ μηδέπω μηδεμίαν ἐνέργειαν τοῦ ζῴου βεβλάφθαι σαφῶς. ὅσον δ᾿ οὖν μεταξὺ τοῦ τ᾿ ἄκρως ἐνεργεῖν καὶ τοῦ βεβλάφθαι σαφῶς ἐνέργειαν ὑπάρχει, τοσοῦτον καὶ τῆς ὑγιείας τὸ πλάτος ἐστὶ καὶ τῆς κατ᾿ αὐτὴν δυσκρασίας. τούτῳ δ᾿ ἐφεξῆς ἐστιν ἡ νοσώδης δυσκρασία, ὅταν γε διὰ δυσκρασίαν νοσῇ (1.610K) τὸ ζῷον· οὐ γὰρ δὴ διὰ ταύτην γε μόνην ἀλλὰ καὶ κατ᾿ ἄλλας διαθέσεις οὐκ ὀλίγας, ὑπὲρ ὧν ἐν τοῖς περὶ τῆς τῶν νοσημάτων διαφορᾶς λογισμοῖς ἐπὶ πλέον εἰρήσεται.

mixed, but the healthy but badly mixed state only a little. It is not possible to define degree here by measure and weight; a sufficient proof of the healthy bad mixture is for no function of the creature to suffer as yet any clear impairment. The range between peak functioning and being clearly injured in function is the latitude between health and the bad mixture itself. Next after the healthy bad mixture is the sick bad mixture, whenever **(1.610K)** the animal is diseased because of a bad mixture (though it might not be sick because of this alone, but rather with respect to many other conditions, which will be laid out more fully in my work concerning the differences of diseases).

4

Nourishing the Body

In Galen's tripartite bodily system, blood begins its journey when it is part of the "concoction" process in the liver. Ingested food is a fundamental part of this process, directly affecting the body's internal balance and providing a mechanism by which the balance can be therapeutically restored in the setting of ill health. Treatises on diet classify foods and drinks into groups based on their own qualities, whether they are wet, dry, hot, cold, or a combination. Many of Galen's recommendations would not pass muster with a modern dietician—for example, his prohibitions against fresh fruit— but may have been sensible in world without reliably clean drinking water, effective waste

disposal systems, or consistently safe means of food preservation. Of interest to modern readers, the chosen excerpts discuss in general terms how food affects health, in a way that, theoretical considerations aside, speaks to a modern interest in the role of food in the promotion and maintenance of wellness.

On the Properties of Foods

"On the Properties of Foods" provides extensive classification of foods according to fundamental qualities, as well as other attributes, including

taste and ease of digestion. The treatise was probably written around 180 CE. Of more general interest, the text also discusses the eating habits of different groups of people living around the Roman Empire (but I have not included those excerpts here). Deeply rooted in Galen's humoral theory, the recommendations in this text would, on the whole, not be medically relevant for modern readers. There are, however, a few sections that are analogous to our current perspective on the importance of foods' characteristics for maintaining and improving health.

(**6.453.2K**) Περὶ τῶν ἐν ταῖς τροφαῖς δυνάμεων οὐκ ὀλίγοι τῶν ἀρίστων ἰατρῶν ἔγραψαν ἐν πολλῇ σπουδῇ θέμενοι τὴν θεωρίαν, ἐπειδὴ χρησιμωτάτη σχεδὸν ἁπασῶν τῶν κατὰ τὴν ἰατρικήν ἐστι· τοῖς μὲν γὰρ ἄλλοις βοηθήμασιν οὐκ ἐν παντὶ καιρῷ χρώμεθα, τροφῆς δὲ χωρὶς οὐχ οἷόν τε ζῆν οὔθ᾽ ὑγιαίνοντας οὔτε νοσοῦντας. εἰκότως οὖν ἐσπούδασαν οἱ πλεῖστοι τῶν ἀρίστων ἰατρῶν ἀκριβῶς ἐπισκέψασθαι τὰς ἐν αὐτῇ δυνάμεις, οἱ μὲν ἐκ τῆς πείρας (**6.454K**) μόνης ἐγνῶσθαί σφισι φάσκοντες αὐτάς, οἱ δὲ καὶ λογισμῷ προσχρῆσθαι βουλόμενοι, τινὲς δὲ καὶ τὸ πλεῖστον αὐτῷ νέμοντες.

(6.453.2K) Not a few of the best physicians have written about the capacities of food, establishing the theory with great diligence, since it is nearly the most useful of all the theories related to medicine. For although we might not use other remedies in every situation, without food, it is not possible to live, whether we are healthy or sick. Reasonably, then, most of the best doctors have endeavored to examine precisely the capacities **(6.454K)** within food, some on the one hand maintaining that they know about these capacities through trial and error alone, others wishing to avail themselves of reasoning, with some even allotting to it the greatest importance.

Foods have different characteristics, and these characteristics affect how they pass through our bodies. Physical activity can also impact digestion.

(6.464.15K) φαίνεται δὲ ταῦτα ταχεῖαν ἢ βραδεῖαν
(6.465K) ἔχοντα τὴν διέξοδον ἤτοι διὰ τὴν ἐξ ἀρχῆς
ἡμῶν φύσιν ἢ διὰ τὴν ἐπίκτητον διάθεσιν τῆς γα-
στρὸς ἢ διὰ τὴν οἰκείαν οὐσίαν. οἰκείαν δ᾽ οὐσίαν
λέγω τῶν ἐσθιομένων τε καὶ πινομένων, ἐπειδὴ τινὰ
μὲν αὐτῶν ἐστιν ὑγρά, τινὰ δὲ ξηρά, καὶ τινὰ μὲν γλίσχρα, τινὰ δ᾽ εὔθρυπτά τε καὶ εὐδιαίρετα, καὶ τινὰ
μὲν δριμύτητας ἐν ἑαυτοῖς ἔχοντα, τινὰ δ᾽ ὀξύτητας
ἢ πικρότητας ἢ γλυκύτητας ἢ ἁλυκότητας ἢ αὐστη-
ρότητας ἢ στρυφνότητας ἤ τινας ἔξωθεν τούτων φαρ-
μακώδεις δυνάμεις ὁμογενεῖς ταῖς τῶν καθαιρόντων
φαρμάκων. ἀτράφαξυς μὲν γὰρ καὶ βλίτον καὶ μα-
λάχη καὶ κολοκύνθη διὰ τὸ γλίσχρα τε εἶναι καὶ
ὑγρὰ θᾶττον τῶν μὴ τοιούτων ὑπέρχεται καὶ μάλιστα τοῖς περιπατοῦσιν ἡσύχως μετὰ τὴν προσφορὰν
αὐτῶν ἐπ᾽ ἐδάφους εἴκοντος μετρίως· ὀλισθαίνει
γὰρ ἐν τῷ κατασείεσθαι μᾶλλον ἢ εἴ τις ἀτρεμίζει
κατακείμενος.

(6.464.15K) And it seems that these foods have either a swift or a slow (6.465K) passage, either because of our congenital nature, or because of a subsequently acquired condition of the stomach, or its intrinsic essence. I speak of the "intrinsic essence" of the things eaten and drunk because some are moist, some are dry, some are sticky, some are easily broken up and easily divided, and some have an essential pungency, some are acid, bitter, sweet, salty, harsh, or sour, or have pharmacological properties like those of purgative drugs. For example, mountain spinach, purple amaranth, mallow, and the round gourd, because they are sticky and moist, pass more quickly than plants that lack these properties, especially in people who, after eating, take a gentle stroll (since the food glides along in one who exerts himself more so than in one who lies unmoving).

(**6.467.14K**) καὶ τοῦτ᾽ εἶναι δοκεῖ τισι τὸ ὑφ᾽ Ἱππο-
κράτους εἰρημένον· "ἐν τροφῇ φαρμακείη ἄριστον."
τοῖς δ᾽ οὐχ οὕτω μόνον ἔδοξεν ἀκούειν, ἀλλὰ κἀπ᾽
ἐκείνων (**6.468K**) ὁ λόγος εἰρῆσθαι δύναται τῶν
οὔτε θρεπτικήν τινα τοῦ ζῴου δύναμιν ἐχόντων

Some foods are purgative, inducing vomiting or rapid bowel movements. It is important to distinguish between foods that reliably have these pharmacological properties, and those foods that are only nutritive. The excerpt here also includes some of Galen's thoughts on restoring internal balance through selection of foodstuffs appropriate to an individual's own particular constitution and mixture. Of course, most physicians no longer subscribe to humoral theories, but dietary recommendations for particular illnesses are still very much part of therapeutic plans.

(6.467.14K) This also seems to be what was stated by Hippocrates: "In food are the best medications."[32] So, it is advisable to heed this statement in reference not only to these things, but also to those foods (6.468K) that do not have any nourishing or purgative capacity for a creature. For he also says that they often

ἐδεσμάτων οὔτε καθαρτικήν. καὶ γὰρ καὶ ταῦτά
φασιν οὐχ ὡς τροφὰς μόνον ἐνεργεῖν πολλάκις, ἀλλὰ
καὶ ὡς φάρμακα, θερμαίνοντα καὶ ψύχοντα καὶ ξη-
ραίνοντα καὶ ὑγραίνοντα σαφῶς ἡμᾶς· ὡς ὅταν γε
μηδέν τι τούτων ἐνεργῇ περὶ τὸ σῶμα τἀνθρώπου,
τρέφῃ δὲ μόνον αὐτό, τηνικαῦτα τὸν φαρμάκου
λόγον οὐχ ἕξει. ὀλίγιστα μὲν οὖν ἐδέσματα τοιαῦτ᾽
ἐστίν· ἄττα δ᾽ ἂν ᾖ, ταῦτα μόνον τὸν τῆς τροφῆς
ἔχει λόγον ἀκριβῆ χωρὶς τοῦ μεταβάλλειν τὸ σῶμα
τοῦ προσενεγκαμένου κατὰ ποιότητα· τὸ μὲν γὰρ
θερμανθὲν ἢ ψυχθὲν ἢ ξηρανθὲν ἢ ὑγρανθὲν ὑπήλλα-
κται κατὰ ποιότητα, τὸ δ᾽ ἐκ τῶν σιτίων ὄγκον οὐ-
σίας ὁμοίας τῷ διαφορηθέντι προσλαβὸν ὡς ὑπὸ
τροφῶν μόνων αὐτῶν ὠφέλεῖται.

τὰ τοίνυν μέσα ταῖς κράσεσιν οὐδεμίαν ἐπικρατοῦ-
σαν ἔχοντα ποιότητα τροφαὶ μόνον εἰσίν, οὐ φάρμακα, μήθ᾽ ὑπάγοντα γαστέρα μήτ᾽ ἐπέχοντα μήτε

function not only as nourishment, but also as medications, since they clearly have heating, cooling, drying, or moistening effects on us. As a result, whenever one of these is not acting on the human body, only nourishing it, then at that time it will not be considered a medication. Such foods as these are very few, but whatever they are, they will be precisely considered nourishment alone without changing the body of the person eating, with respect to the quality [of that body]. For a substance that was warmed, cooled, dried, or moistened undergoes a change in quality, but the body that has taken from food a mass of substance equal to what had been dispersed benefits from this food as nourishment only.

Thus, things that are at the mean in their mixture, without a prevailing quality, are food alone, not medications, neither purging or restraining

HOW TO BE HEALTHY

ῥωννύντα μήτ' ἐκλύοντα στόμαχον, ὥσπερ **(6.469K)**
γε μήθ' ἱδρῶτας ἢ οὖρα κινοῦντα μήτ' ἄλλην τινὰ διάθεσιν ἐν τῷ σώματι ποιοῦντα κατὰ θερμότητα καὶ
ψυχρότητα καὶ ξηρότητα καὶ ὑγρότητα, διαφυλάτ-
τοντα δὲ πάντῃ τὸ τοῦ τρεφομένου ζῴου σῶμα
τοιοῦτον, ὁποῖον παρέλαβεν. ἀλλὰ κἀνταῦθα διορι-
σμός τίς ἐστι χρησιμώτατος οὐδ' αὐτὸς ὑπὸ τοῦ Διο-
κλέους εἰρημένος, ὥσπερ οὐδὲ τῶν ἄλλων τις, ὅσους
μέχρι τοῦδε διῆλθον.

εἰ μὲν γὰρ ἀκριβῶς μέσον εἴη τῇ κράσει τὸ σῶμα
τἀνθρώπου, φυλάττοιτ' ἂν ὑπὸ τῆς μέσης τῇ κράσει
τροφῆς ἐν τῇ παρούσῃ καταστάσει· εἰ δ' ἤτοι θερ-
μότερον ἢ ψυχρότερον ἢ ξηρότερον ἢ ὑγρότερον εἴη,
τούτῳ τὰ μέσα τῇ κράσει σιτία τε καὶ ποτὰ κακῶς
ἄν τις διδοίη. μεταβάλλεσθαι γὰρ ἕκαστον χρὴ τῶν

the belly, nor tightening or relaxing the stomach. In like manner **(6.469K)**, they do not promote sweating or urination, or create any other condition in the body with regard to warming, cooling, drying, and moistening, but rather in every respect preserve the body of the creature that is nourished in the same condition as it was when it ingested them. But here a certain distinction is very useful, though not the one discussed by Diocles (just as none of the other distinctions I have discussed up to this point have been useful).

If a human body were exactly at the mean in mixture, it would be preserved in the existing state by food that is at the mean in mixture. If the body were warmer, colder, drier, or wetter, however, then if someone should give it food and drink that were at the mean in mixture, he would be doing harm. For each of these sorts of bodies needs to be moved toward its opposite

τοιούτων σωμάτων ἐπὶ τοὐναντίον, εἰς ὅσον ἀπεχώ-
ρησε τῆς ἀκριβῶς μέσης καταστάσεως· ἔσται δὲ
τοῦτο διὰ τῶν ἐναντίων τῇ παρούσῃ δυσκρασίᾳ. τὰ
δ᾽ ἐναντία τὴν ἴσην ἀφέστηκε τοῦ μέσου διάστασιν
ἐφ᾽ ἑκάτερα καθ᾽ ἑκατέραν ἀντίθεσιν, ὥστ᾽, ἐὰν μὲν
ἀριθμοῖς, εἰ τύχοι, τρισὶν ἀπὸ τῆς εὐκράτου τε καὶ
μέσης (6.470K) καταστάσεως ἀποχωρήσῃ τὸ σῶμα
πρὸς τὴν θερμοτέραν, τοσούτοις χρῆναι καὶ τὸ σιτίον
ἀφεστάναι τοῦ μέσου τῇ κράσει πρὸς τὸ ψυχρότερον,
ἐὰν δ᾽ ἐφ᾽ ὑγρότητα τέτταρσιν ἀριθμοῖς ἀποστῇ,
τοῖς ἴσοις δεῖν εἶναι ξηρότερον τοῦ συμμέτρου.

to the same extent as it departs from its precisely mean state, and this change will come about through things opposite to the existing bad mixture. The opposites stand an equal distance from the mean, toward each opposite according to the respective contraries. Consequently, if a body is three units away from the well-mixed, mean **(6.470K)** state in the direction of a warmer state, then food for this body would need to stand at the same interval away from the mean in mixture in the direction of the colder condition; or, if the body were four units toward wetness, then the food should be drier than the good balance by an equal number of units.[33]

5

Definitions of Health and Disease

Definitions of health and disease were of fundamental importance for Galen. Without precise definitions, he notes, one cannot build a strong, useful theoretical system. Clear terminology yields a well-defined classification scheme, which in turn can provide insight into issues of causality, which themselves suggest treatment options. Galen devotes several long treatises to definitions of health and disease, written not only to outline his own views but also to refute definitions and theories propounded by rival physicians (living and deceased). The following excerpts were chosen because they provide insight into how Galen thought about disease and because they engage

productively and incisively with the idea of what is "normal." Of the five sections included in this book, this contains excerpts that are most philosophical and theoretical—and in many respects, the most difficult to read.

I have included them, despite their difficulty, because I feel that they are very relevant for modern conceptions of health and disease. As our own medical technologies provide voluminously increased quantities of data about any one person, down to that person's DNA, and then combine one person's data with those of millions of other people in order to situate people on spectra of disease processes, we become more aware of the complications associated with the idea of "normal." For example, accumulation of calcium in a person's arteries is somewhat expected for someone in her eighties but is not normal for someone in her twenties. We would call atherosclerotic vascular disease

pathological under any circumstances, in that it predisposes patients to bad outcomes, but it is a "normal" part of human aging, in that most people demonstrate calcifications in their arteries, to varying degrees, as they age. However, the amount and location of calcifications, the age at which they begin to accumulate, and the nature of associated symptoms affect how pathological we consider them to be. Galen is careful to relate his understanding of health and disease to a concept of functionality, not unlike how modern physicians think about quality of life as the ability of patients to achieve specific goals that matter to them.

We should also recognize that totalizing concepts of health and disease might similarly be understood more granularly. For example, someone might be completely healthy except for a broken arm. Another person with a benign liver tumor that causes mild laboratory

abnormalities but no other problems might also be said to be healthy, except for a problem in one specific organ. If that liver tumor were malignant, then the health of the other parts of a patient's body would be of paramount concern in discussions regarding suitability for a liver transplant. Patients can have acute exacerbations of chronic conditions, as is commonly seen in asthma or in multiple sclerosis, for example. They can have chronic conditions that predispose them to other illnesses, or to more severe forms of other illnesses, such as osteomyelitis in the setting of diabetes.

As shown in the included texts, Galen, too, noticed that health and disease may be defined in relative terms, with respect to an individual patient's baseline condition, with respect to age, and with respect to body part (among other categories). Although the precise classification of named diseases did not play the same founda-

tional role for Galen as it does for a modern physician, clear definitions of health and disease facilitated characterization of symptoms and internal derangements. Such characterization was, for Galen, a necessary precursor to the restoration of balance that constituted treatment. In these passages, Galen draws on not only his experience as a physician, but also his deep knowledge of philosophy, epistemology, and logic.

On Hygiene

In this additional section of "On Hygiene," which appears at the outset of that treatise (before the sections on exercise), Galen notes that hygiene is age dependent and that the methods used to maintain a good condition of the body will, therefore, vary as the body changes with age. Galen here makes intriguing (and, to us, very modern) arguments about health as a range

(6.13.8K) Ἐπὶ τούτοις ὑποκειμένοις ἀρκτέον ἂν εἴη ἐνθένδε τῆς ὑγιεινῆς πραγματείας. ἐπειδὴ συμμετρία τίς ἐστιν ἡ ὑγεία, συμμετρία δὲ πᾶσα κατὰ διττὸν ἀποτελεῖται καὶ λέγεται τρόπον, ποτὲ μὲν εἰς ἄκρον ἥκουσα καὶ ὄντως οὖσα συμμετρία, ποτὲ δὲ ἀπολειπομένη βραχύ τι τῆς ἀκριβείας, εἴη ἂν καὶ ἡ ὑγιεινὴ

or a spectrum, emphasizing that health involves being able to do what you want to do, in an age-appropriate way. As he describes it, this position contrasts with that of some of his ideological opponents, who, he says, assert that health is a strictly defined state of perfect physical fitness. Some of the sections defining health as a spectrum are included here in translation.

INDIVIDUALIZED DEFINITIONS
OF HEALTH AND DISEASE

(6.13.8K) On these assumptions one must begin the systematic study of hygiene from here. Because health is a certain good balance,[34] and because every good balance is produced and spoken of in two ways—in one sense, of reaching a peak and truly being a good balance, and in the other sense, of falling somewhat short in precision—hygiene would also be a certain good balance in two senses: the one that is precise,

συμμετρία διττή τις· ἡ μὲν γὰρ ἀκριβής τε καὶ ἀρί-
στη καὶ τελέα καὶ ἄκρα, ἡ δὲ ἀπολειπομένη μὲν
ταύτης, οὐ μὴν ἤδη γέ πω τοσούτῳ, ὡς λυπεῖσθαι τὸ
ζῷον. ἔστι δὲ κἀνταῦθα λογική τις μᾶλλον **(6.14K)** ἢ
κατὰ τὴν χρείαν τῆς τέχνης ζήτησις, οὐ συγχωρού-
ντων ἐνίων ἕτερον ἑτέρου μᾶλλον ὑγιαίνειν οὐδ᾽ εἶναι
πλάτος ἱκανὸν ἐν τῇ διαθέσει τοῦ σώματος, ἣν ὑγίαν
ὀνομάζομεν, ἀλλ᾽ ἕν τι καὶ ἀπηκριβωμένον οὖσαν
αὐτὴν ἄτμητον εἰς τὸ μᾶλλόν τε καὶ ἧττον ὑπάρχειν.
ἐμοὶ δὲ ὥσπερ τὸ λευκὸν σῶμα τὸ μὲν ἧττον φαίνεται λευκὸν εἶναι, τὸ δὲ μᾶλλον, οὕτω καὶ τὸ ὑγιαῖνον
ἧττόν τε καὶ μᾶλλον εἶναι δοκεῖ τοιοῦτον.

διττὴ δὲ ἀπόδειξις τοῦ λόγου· μία μὲν ἐκ τῆς κατὰ
τὰς ἡλικίας μεταπτώσεως· ἀφ᾽ οὗ γὰρ ἂν ἀποκυηθῇ
τὸ ζῷον, ἀεὶ μεταβάλλειν ἀναγκαῖον αὐτοῦ τὴν κρᾶσιν, ὡς ἔμπροσθεν ἐδείκνυμεν· ὥστ᾽, εἴπερ ἐν μὲν τῷ

best, complete, and consummate, and the other that falls short of it, but not yet to such a point that the animal is harmed. And there is a question here too that is somewhat more theoretical than **(6.14K)** of practical relevance to the art, since some people do not allow that one person is healthier than another, or that bodily condition exists along a considerable latitude, which we call health. Instead, these people say that health is one single and very precise thing that cannot be subdivided into "more healthy" or "less healthy." But just as in the case of a white body, one seems to me to be less white and another more white,[35] so too the healthy body seems to me to be more or less healthy.

There are two proofs for this argument. First, on the basis of a change of phase of life: From whenever an animal is born, it necessarily continuously changes in its mixture, as I have pointed out previously, so that if health lies in a

ποιῷ τῆς κράσεως ἡ ὑγεία, τὸ ποιὸν δ᾽ οὐ μένει
ταὐτόν, οὐδὲ τὴν ὑγείαν ἐγχωρεῖ τὴν αὐτὴν φυλάτ-
τεσθαι. δευτέρα δ᾽ ἀπόδειξις ἐκ τῆς κατὰ τὰς ἐνεργείας διαφορᾶς· οὔτε γὰρ τοῖς ὀφθαλμοῖς ὡσαύτως
ἅπαντες οἱ ὑγιαίνοντες ὁρῶσιν (ἀλλ᾽ οἱ μὲν μᾶλλον,
οἱ δ᾽ ἧττον), οὔτε τοῖς ὠσὶν ὁμοίως ἀκούουσιν (ἀλλὰ
κἀνταῦθα πάμπολυ τὸ μᾶλλόν [6.15K] τε καὶ ἧττον),
οὐ μὴν οὐδὲ τοῖς σκέλεσιν ὡσαύτως θέουσιν οὐδὲ
ἀντιλαμβάνονται ταῖς χερσὶν οὐδὲ τοῖς ἄλλοις ἅπασιν ὀργάνοις ὡσαύτως ἐνεργοῦσιν, ἀλλ᾽ ὁ μέν τις
βέλτιον, ὁ δὲ χεῖρον. εἴπερ οὖν αἱ διαφοραὶ τῶν ἐνεργειῶν ταῖς τῶν κράσεων διαφοραῖς ἀκολουθοῦσιν,
ἀνάγκη τοσαύτας εἶναι τὰς τῶν κράσεων διαφοράς,
ὅσαιπέρ εἰσι καὶ αἱ τῶν ἐνεργειῶν.

εἰ δὲ μὴ κράσεων ἐθέλοι τις λέγειν, ἀλλὰ κατασκευῶν, ἵν᾽ ἐπὶ πάσαις ταῖς αἱρέσεσιν ὁ λόγος

certain kind of mixture, and if the quality of the mixture does not remain the same, then it is not possible that health be preserved as always the same. The second proof of the argument is based on the difference in functions. All healthy people do not see in the same way with their eyes (some see better, and some see worse), nor do they hear similarly with their ears (but here too some hear very well, [6.15K] others less so), nor do they run similarly with their legs or grasp similarly with their hands, nor do they function similarly with respect to all their other organs, but one better, another worse. If, then, differences in functions follow the differences in mixtures, it is necessary that there be as many differences of mixtures as there are also of functions.

If someone should not wish to speak of "mixtures" but would rather say differences of "constitutions" in order that the argument

ἐκτείνοιτο, συμπεραίνοιτ' ἂν ὡσαύτως. συμμετρία γὰρ δή τις ἡ ὑγεία κατὰ πάσας ἐστὶ τὰς αἱρέσεις, ἀλλὰ καθ' ἡμᾶς μὲν ὑγροῦ καὶ ξηροῦ καὶ θερμοῦ καὶ ψυχροῦ, κατ' ἄλλους δὲ ὄγκων καὶ πόρων, κατ' ἄλλους δὲ ἀτόμων ἢ ἀνάρμων ἢ ἀμερῶν ἢ ὁμοιομερῶν ἢ ἀνομοιομερῶν ἢ ὅτου δὴ τῶν πρώτων στοιχείων, ἀλλὰ κατὰ πάντας γε διὰ τὴν συμμετρίαν αὐτῶν ἐνεργοῦμεν τοῖς μορίοις. εἴπερ οὖν διαφόρως ἐνεργοῦμεν, διάφορός ἐστι καὶ ἡ καθ' ἕκαστον συμμετρία τῶν στοιχείων, ἥπερ ἦν ἡ ὑγεία.

καὶ μὴν καὶ χωρὶς τοῦ τῶν στοιχείων μνημονεύειν **(6.16K)** ὧδ' ἂν ὁ λόγος ἐρωτηθείη. εἴπερ ταῖς

should extend to all the medical sects, he would draw similar conclusions.[36] For health is indeed some good balance, according to all the medical sects. According to us, it is a good balance among the wet, the dry, the hot, and the cold; according to others, a good balance among corpuscles and pores; and to still others, a good balance among things that are indivisible, or without joints, or without parts, or composed of uniform parts, or composed of nonuniform parts, or of some one or other primary element. But according to everyone, it is owing to a good balance of these things that we function in our parts. So, if we then function in different ways, the good balance of each individual's elements is also different—and this is the very thing that we said health was.

And what is more, even without making reference **(6.16K)** to the elements, the argument could be propounded in the following way: if

κατασκευαῖς τῶν μορίων ἀκολουθοῦσιν αἱ ἐνέργειαι, ὅσαιπερ ἂν ὦσιν ἐν ταῖς ἐνεργείαις αἱ διαφοραί, τοσαῦται κἂν ταῖς κατασκευαῖς ἔσονται· ἀλλὰ μὴν ἀκολουθοῦσιν ταῖς κατασκευαῖς αἱ ἐνέργειαι· ἀναγκαῖον ἄρα τοσαύτας εἶναι τῶν κατασκευῶν τὰς διαφοράς, ὅσαιπερ καὶ αἱ τῶν ἐνεργειῶν. εἰσὶ δὲ αἱ τῶν ἐνεργειῶν πάμπολλαι· τινες ἄρα καὶ τῶν κατασκευῶν εἰσιν. εἴπερ οὖν ἐν ἅπασι τοῖς ὑγιαίνουσιν αἱ κατασκευαὶ τῶν μορίων ὑπάρχουσι σύμμετροι, διάφοροι δέ εἰσιν αἱ κατασκευαί, διότι καὶ αἱ ἐνέργειαι διάφοροι, πάμπολλαί τινες ἄρα συμμετρίαι τῶν κατασκευῶν ἔσονται, ὥστε καὶ ὑγεῖαι πάμπολλαι.

καὶ μὴν εἰ διαφέρουσιν ἀλλήλων αἱ κατὰ μέρος ὑγεῖαι, ἤτοι κατὰ τὸ κοινὸν ἐν ἁπάσαις εἶδος (ἀφ' οὗπερ ὑγεῖαι λέγονται), διοίσουσιν ἢ κατὰ τὸ μᾶλλόν

the functions follow the constitutions of the parts, then however many differences there are in the functions, so many will be the differences also in constitutions. Yet the functions do in fact follow the constitutions, so it is necessary that the differences of the constitutions be so many as are also the differences of the functions. There are many differences in functions, so there are certain differences of constitutions, too. So, if in all healthy people the constitutions of the parts are well balanced, but their constitutions are different, such that their functions are also different, then there will be a great many kinds of good balances of constitutions, and so, too, many healthy states.

But if these healthy states differ in particulars from one another, then either they will differ among all in respect of a common form (on the basis of which they are said to be healthy), or they differ from one another to a greater or

τε καὶ ἧττον ἀλλήλων διαφέρουσιν· ἀλλὰ μὴν οὐ κατὰ
τὸ κοινὸν <εἶδος>· ἀδιάφοροι γάρ εἰσιν αἱ ὑγεῖαι· κατὰ
τὸ μᾶλλον ἄρα καὶ ἧττον ἀλλήλων διαφέρουσιν.
ὥσπερ γὰρ ἡ ἐν τῇ χιόνι λευκότης τῆς ἐν (6.17K) τῷ
γάλακτι λευκότητος, ᾗ μὲν λευκόν ἐστιν, οὐ διαφέρει,
τῷ μᾶλλον δὲ καὶ ἧττον διαφέρει, τὸν αὐτὸν δὴ τρόπον ἡ ἐν τῷ Ἀχιλλεῖ, φέρε εἰπεῖν, ὑγεία τῆς ἐν τῷ
Θερσίτῃ ὑγείας, καθ᾽ ὅσον μὲν ὑγεία, ταὐτόν ἐστιν,
ἑτέρῳ δέ τινι διάφορος· καὶ τοῦτο τὸ ἕτερον οὐδὲν
ἄλλο ἐστὶν ἢ τὸ μᾶλλόν τε καὶ ἧττον. οὔτε γὰρ ὡς οὐ
διαφερόντως ἐνεργοῦμεν ἅπαντες ἔνεστιν εἰπεῖν οὔθ᾽
ὡς δι᾽ ἄλλο τι τὴν ἀνισότητα ταύτην ἔχομεν ἢ διὰ τὴν
κατασκευήν, ἀφ᾽ ἧς ἐνεργοῦμεν. εἰ δέ τις φήσει μόνους μὲν τοὺς ἅπασι τοῖς μορίοις ἄκρως ἐνεργοῦντας
ὑγιαίνειν, ἡμᾶς δὲ τοὺς ἄλλους, ὅσοι χεῖρον ἐκείνων

lesser degree. But, they will not differ in respect
to a common form, because healthy states are
not different. They therefore differ more or less
from one another. For just as the whiteness of
snow does not differ from **(6.17K)** the whiteness
of milk, insofar as it is white, but differs in being
more or less white, in the same way, the health
of Achilles, for example, is the same as the
health of Thersites, insofar as it is health, but is
different in some other way — and this other way
in which it differs is nothing other than being
of a greater or lesser degree. For it is impossible
to say that we all do not differ in our functions
or that we possess this inequality for any other
reason than for the constitution on the basis of
which we function. If someone will say that
only those at peak function in all their parts are
healthy, and that the rest of us who are inferior
to them are not healthy, he should know that
he is totally overturning the assumption of the

ἔχομεν, οὐχ ὑγιαίνειν, ἴστω συμπάσης οὗτος τῆς ὑγιεινῆς πραγματείας ἀνατρέπων τὴν ὑπόθεσιν. εἰ γὰρ δὴ τὸ φυλάττειν ἣν παρελάβομεν ὑγείαν ὁ σκοπός ἐστιν αὐτῆς, οὐδεὶς δὲ ἡμῶν ὑγιαίνει, πρόδηλον, ὡς ἐπ' οὐδενὸς ἐνεργοῦσαν ἕξομεν ἣν νῦν συστῆσαι βουλόμεθα τέχνην ὑγιεινήν· οὐκοῦν οὐδὲ ζητητέον αὐτήν, ἀλλὰ σιωπητέον τε καὶ **(6.18K)** καταπαυστέον ἤδη τὸν λόγον. ἁπάσας οὖν ἐκκόπτει τὰς τοιαύτας ἀπορίας ἡ τοῦ ἀληθοῦς γνῶσις· οὐ γὰρ ἡ τελεία μόνον ἥτις ἐστὶν ἄτμητος ὑγεία λέγεταί τε καὶ ἔστιν, ἀλλὰ καὶ ἡ τῆσδε μὲν ἀποδέουσα, μηδέπω δὲ τῆς χρείας ἐκπεπτωκυῖα.

χρήζομεν γὰρ ἅπαντες ἄνθρωποι τῆς ὑγείας εἴς τε τὰς κατὰ τὸν βίον ἐνεργείας, ἃς ἐμποδίζουσί τε ἢ διακόπτουσι καὶ καταπαύουσιν αἱ νόσοι, καὶ προσέτι τῆς ἀνοχλησίας ἕνεκεν· ὀχλούμεθα γὰρ ἐν ταῖς ὀδύναις οὐ σμικρά. τὴν δὲ τοιαύτην κατάστασιν, ἐν ᾗ

systematic study of hygiene. For if the aim of hygiene is the preservation of the health that we possess, but none of us is healthy, it is obvious that the hygienic art that we now want to establish will not be functional for anyone, and consequently that we should not even pursue it, but instead keep our silence and **(6.18K)** cease our discussion immediately. Recognition of the truth makes an end of all such difficulties, for it is the case that not only the perfect and indivisible health is spoken about and exists, but also the health that falls short of perfect health but has not yet departed from its utility.

We humans, all of us, desire health for the activities of life, which sicknesses interfere with, or interrupt and stop entirely. Besides this, health is desired for the sake of freedom from disturbance. For we are disturbed to no little degree by pains. We call "health" that sort of state in which we are neither in pain nor hindered

μήτε ὀδυνώμεθα μήτε ἐν ταῖς κατὰ τὸν βίον ἐνεργείαις ἐμποδιζόμεθα, καλοῦμεν ὑγείαν, ἣν εἴ τις
ἑτέρῳ προσαγορεύειν ὀνόματι βούλεται, πλέον οὐδὲν
ἐκ τούτων σχήσει, καθάπερ οὖν οὐδ' οἱ τὴν 'ἀει-
πάθειαν' εἰσάγοντες. εἰ μὲν γὰρ διὰ τοῦτ' εἰσῆγον
αὐτήν, ὅτι πᾶν σῶμα γεννητόν, ὥσπερ τὰς τῆς γενέ-
σεως αἰτίας, οὕτω καὶ τὰς τῆς φθορᾶς ἔχει συμφύτους
ἐξ ἀρχῆς, ὡς ἡμεῖς ἐπεδείξαμεν ἔμπροσθεν, ἐπῃνοῦ-
μεν ἂν αὐτούς, ὡς ἀληθῆ τε ἅμα καὶ παλαιὰ πρε-
σβεύοντας δόγματα. ἐπειδὴ δὲ ὁμοειδῆ τὴν τῶν
ὑγιαινόντων σωμάτων κατάστασιν εἶναι (6.19K)
βούλονται τοῖς τῶν νοσούντων, οὐκέτ' ἐπαινοῦμεν
οὐδὲ ἀποδεχόμεθα τὸ δόγμα· βέλτιον γὰρ ἦν μακρῷ
πλάτος ὑποθέσθαι συχνὸν ἔχειν τὴν ὑγείαν ἤπερ ἅπαντας ἡμᾶς ἀπαύστῳ νοσήματι συνέχεσθαι.

καὶ γὰρ εἰ τὰ σπέρματα τῶν νόσων ἐνυπάρχειν
ἡμῖν φασιν, ἀλλά τοι συγχωροῦσί γε καὶ αὐτοὶ διὰ
τὴν σμικρότητα τὴν αἴσθησιν ἡμῶν ἐκφεύγειν αὐτά.

with respect to the activities of life. If someone wishes to call this state by another name, he will not actually achieve anything more by this, just as those who introduce the word "permanent affection" do not.[37] If, however, they introduce the term for this reason, that every generated body, just as it has congenital causes of growth, so also has congenital causes of decay right from the beginning, as we pointed out earlier, then we would commend them for giving precedence to true and also ancient doctrines. But since they want the states of healthy bodies **(6.19K)** to be similar to those of people who are sick, we can no longer commend them nor accept their doctrine. It is better to assume that health has a wide latitude than to say that we are all afflicted by unceasing disease.

Although they say to us that the seeds of sickness are inside of us, nevertheless these same people also concede that the seeds escape our

ἔστω τοίνυν, εἰ βούλονται, καὶ ὀδυνηρά τις ἐν ἡμῖν
διάθεσις, ἀλλ' οὕτω σμικρὰ καὶ ἀναίσθητος, ὡς μὴ
λυπεῖν τοὺς ἔχοντας. ἔστωσαν, εἰ βούλονται καὶ πυ-
ρετοί, ἀλλ' οὕτω σμικροί, ὡς μήτ' αἴσθησιν ἀπ' αὐτῶν
ἡμῖν γίνεσθαι μηδεμίαν ἐξεῖναί τε καὶ πολιτεύεσθαι
καὶ λούεσθαι καὶ πίνειν ἐσθίειν τε καὶ τἄλλα πράττειν, ὧν δεόμεθα.

τὸ γὰρ τῆς χρείας ἀπαρεμπόδιστον ὁρίζει μᾶλλον
τὴν ὑγείαν. οὐδὲ γὰρ ἡ τῶν ἐνεργειῶν ἀσθένεια νόσου
γνώρισμά ἐστιν, οὕτως ἁπλῶς εἰποῦσιν, ἀλλὰ ἡ παρὰ
τὴν ἑκάστου φύσιν. ὡς ἅπαντές γε κακῶς ὁρῶμεν, εἰ
τοῖς ἀετοῖς τε καὶ Λυγκεῖ παραβαλλοίμεθα, καὶ δὴ
καὶ ἀκούομεν οὐκ (6.20K) ὀρθῶς, εἰ Μελάμποδι, καὶ
τοῖς ποσὶν ἀρρωστοῦμεν, εἴ τις ἡμᾶς Ἰφίκλῳ παρα-
βάλλοι, καὶ ταῖς χερσίν, εἰ Μίλωνι, καὶ καθ' ἕκαστον

notice on account of their small size.[38] Well then, let there also be posited, if they so wish, a certain painful condition within us, but one so tiny and imperceptible that we are not able to experience discomfort. Let them posit too, if they wish, fevers, but ones so small that there exists no perception of them to us and it is possible for us to go about our affairs, bathe, drink, eat, and do the other things we want.

Unimpeded activity is what actually defines health. Nor is weakness of functions a hallmark of sickness, if we were to say this without qualification, but only the kind of weakness that is contrary to the nature of each individual. Thus, all of us have poor sight if we compare ourselves to eagles or to Lynceus, and bad hearing **(6.20K)** if to Melampus; we are lame in our feet if someone should compare us to Iphicles, and in hands if to Milo;[39] and so on through each part we would be considered nearly disabled if we were

δὴ μόριον ἐγγὺς ἂν ἥκειν νομισθείημεν πηρώσεως, εἰ τοῖς πρωτεύσασι κατά τι παραβαλλοίμεθα.

τίς γοῦν ἡμῶν φαύλως ἔχειν οἴεται τῶν ὀφθαλμῶν, εἰ μὴ βλέποι τοὺς ἀπὸ δυοῖν σταδίων μύρμηκας; ἢ τίς τῶν ὤτων, εἰ μὴ κατακούοι τῶν ἀφ' ἑξήκοντα σταδίων; ἀλλ' εἰ ταῦτα τὰ γράμματα, τὰ κατὰ τουτὶ τὸ βιβλίον ἐγγεγραμμένα, μὴ βλέποι τις ὀρθῶς, εὐλόγως οὗτος <ἂν> ἤδη μέμψαιτο τὰς ὄψεις· οὐ μὴν οὐδ' εἰ ταῦτα τέσσαρας ἀποστήσας πήχεις μὴ βλέποι, δικαίως ἂν μέμφοιτο, πλὴν εἰ τῶν οὕτω τις ὀξυωπεστάτων εἴη τὴν φύσιν, ὡς καὶ ταῦτα ἐμβλέπειν. οὕτω γάρ, οἶμαι, καὶ μέμψεται καὶ δικαίως φήσει, ὥσπερ ἅπαντες ἄνθρωποι λέγουσιν, ὡς τόδε τι κατὰ τὸν ἔμπροσθεν χρόνον ἐνεργῶν εἶτα νῦν οὐκ ἐνεργεῖ. τὸν μὲν γὰρ τοιοῦτον ἐν νόσῳ τινὶ φήσομεν ὑπάρχειν, εἴπερ μὴ διὰ γῆρας ταῦτα πάσχοι· (καίτοι καὶ τοῦτο νόσον εἶναι λέγουσιν ἔνιοι).

to compare ourselves those who are preeminent in some respect.

Is there really any of us who would think that he has poor eyes, if he could not see ants half a mile away? Or poor ears, if he could not hear those who are fourteen miles away? Rather, if someone could not properly see the letters written in this book, then he would rightly find fault with his eyes. Nor again, if he could not see the letters from four arms' lengths away would he justly consider his eyes faulty, unless he were one of those people who are extremely sharp eyed by nature such that they can read letters at this distance, too. For he would, I think, in this case find fault with his eyes and justly say, as all do, that although he had been able to do such a thing before, his eyes no longer function this way. Therefore, we say that this kind of person is affected by some sickness unless he should experience these things owing to old age

τοὺς δ᾽ ἄλλους ἅπαντας, οἷς φύσει μήτ᾽ ὀξὺ βλέπειν μήτ᾽ (6.21Κ) ἀκούειν ὑπάρχει μήτε θέειν ὠκέως
ἤ τι τοιοῦτον ἕτερον ἐνεργεῖν ἰσχυρῶς, οὔτε νοσεῖν
οὔθ᾽ ὅλως παρὰ φύσιν ἔχειν ὑποληψόμεθα. πᾶσαι μὲν
γὰρ αἱ νόσοι παρὰ φύσιν, οὐκ ἔχουσι δ᾽ οἱ τοιοῦτοι
παρὰ φύσιν, ὥσπερ οὐδ᾽ οἱ γέροντες. οὔκουν ἁπλῶς
γε τῶν ἐνεργειῶν εὐρωστίᾳ τε καὶ ἀρρωστίᾳ κριτέον
ἐστὶ τοὺς ὑγιαίνοντάς τε καὶ νοσοῦντας, ἀλλὰ τὸ κατὰ
φύσιν μὲν τοῖς ὑγιαίνουσι, τὸ παρὰ φύσιν δὲ τοῖς νο-
σοῦσι προσθετέον, ὡς εἶναι τὴν μὲν ὑγείαν διάθεσιν
κατὰ φύσιν ἐνεργείας ποιητικήν, τὴν δὲ νόσον διάθεσιν παρὰ φύσιν ἐνεργείας βλαπτικήν. οὔτε γὰρ ἡ
κατὰ φύσιν διάθεσις ἤδη καὶ ὑγεία (διάθεσις γάρ τίς
ἐστι κατὰ φύσιν ἥ τε τῶν Αἰγυπτίων μελανότης ἥ τε

(but in fact there are some who do say that old age is also a sickness).

But we will not suppose that all the others who by nature are not able to see or **(6.21K)** to hear acutely, to run swiftly, or to function vigorously in some other such respect are sick or wholly contrary to nature, since all sicknesses are contrary to nature, but such people are not contrary to nature, no more than the elderly are. One must not decide who is healthy and sick simply by the strength or weakness of their functions. Instead, one should apply the concept of "in accordance with nature" to those who are healthy, and the concept of "contrary to nature" to those who are sick, such that health is a condition in accordance with nature that creates function, while sickness is a condition contrary to nature injurious to function. For a condition in accordance with nature is not immediately healthy (for example, the darker

τῶν Κελτῶν λευκότης ἤ τε τῶν Σκυθῶν πυρρότης·
ἀλλ’ οὐδὲν τῶν τοιούτων ὑγείας δηλωτικόν, διότι μηδ’
ἐν χρώμασιν ὅλως ἡ ὑγεία) οὔτ’ εἰ παρὰ φύσιν, ἤδη
καὶ νόσος (ὡς εἴη γ’ ἂν οὕτω νόσος ἥ τ’ ἐξ ἡλίου μελανότης ἥ τ’ ἐκ μακρᾶς σκιατροφίας λευκότης), ἀλλὰ
προσθεῖναι χρὴ τῇ μὲν τῆς (6.22K) ὑγείας ἐννοίᾳ τὸ
λόγον αἰτίας ἔχειν αὐτὴν πρὸς τὴν ἐνέργειαν, τῇ δὲ
τῆς νόσου τὸ καὶ ταύτην τὴν ἐνέργειαν βλάπτειν.

ἀλλὰ περὶ μὲν τούτων ἐν ἑτέροις εἴρηται διὰ
πλειόνων, εἰς δὲ τὰ παρόντα τοσοῦτον ἀποχρήσει
μόνον ἐξ αὐτῶν εἰλῆφθαι, τὸ πλάτος ἱκανὸν εἶναι τῆς
ὑγείας, καὶ μὴ πᾶσιν ἡμῖν ὑπάρχειν ἴσον ἀκριβῶς. εἰ
δέ τῳ δοκεῖ βίαιον εἶναι καὶ τὴν μὴ παντάπασιν

complexion of the Egyptians, the lighter complexion of the Celts, or the reddish complexion of the Scythians is each a certain condition in accordance with nature, but none of these kinds of things is indicative of health, because health does not reside entirely in complexions), nor is a condition contrary to nature immediately a disease (since then a darker complexion from the sun or white skin from an extended period in the shade would be a disease). Rather, we must add to the notion of health **(6.22K)** a causal account in relation to function, and similarly to the notion of disease the fact that it injures this function as well.

But these things have been described extensively in other works. In the present circumstances, it will suffice to go only so far as to draw this conclusion, that there is a considerable latitude in health, and it is not precisely equal for all of us. But if it should seem forced to

ἠκριβωμένην εὐκρασίαν ὅμως ἔτι καὶ αὐτὴν ὀνομά-
ζεσθαι, οὗτος ἀναμνησθήτω τῶν κατὰ τὸν βίον ἁπάντων ὀνομάτων. εὔκρατον οὖν τι καὶ πόμα φαμὲν εἶναι
καὶ βαλανεῖον, οὐ μόνον ὅτι τὸ μὲν ἄλλῳ, τὸ δὲ ἄλλῳ
τοιοῦτόν ἐστιν, ἀλλὰ ὅτι καὶ πρὸς τὸν αὐτὸν ἄνθρωπον ἐν πλάτει τοιοῦτον ὑπάρχει· ἀποστραφέντος γοῦν
τοῦ πίνοντος, ἐμβαλὼν εἰς τὸ ποτήριον ἤτοι θερμὸν
ἢ ψυχρὸν βραχὺ λάθοις ἄν. καίτοι γ', εἴπερ ἦν οὕτως
ἀπηκριβωμένον τὸ εὔκρατον, ὡς ἓν εἶναι καὶ ἄτμητον, οὐκ ἂν ἐπιβαλόντος θερμὸν ἢ ψυχρὸν ἔτι εὔκρατον ἐφαίνετο. κατὰ δὲ τὸν αὐτὸν τρόπον, οὐδ' (6.23K)
εἰ βραχύ τις εἰς τὴν εὔκρατον κολυμβήθραν ἐμβάλ-
λοι ψυχροῦ, διαφθερεῖ παραχρῆμα τὴν εὐκρασίαν
αὐτῆς. οὕτω δὲ καὶ τὸ περιέχον εὔκρατον εἶναί φαμεν,
εἰ καὶ βραχείας ἐφ' ἑκάτερα τροπὰς λαμβάνει. καὶ
τί θαυμαστόν, εἰ τὴν εὐκρασίαν εἰς ἱκανὸν ἐκτεί-
νουσι πλάτος ἅπαντες, ὅπου γε καὶ τὴν ἐν ταῖς λύραις
εὐαρμοστίαν τὴν μὲν ἀκριβεστάτην δήπου μίαν καὶ

anyone that we still call this good mixture "health" even though it is not made entirely precise, let him remember all the senses of "good mixture" that are found in daily life. We say that a drink and a bath are well mixed, not only because it is so for one person or another, but also because even for the same person what is well mixed has latitude—at least, if the one drinking had turned his back, and you added a little something cold or hot into his cup, you could deceive him. Yet, if what is well mixed were made so precise as to be one and indivisible, then it would no longer seem well mixed with the addition of hot or cold. In the same way, if **(6.23K)** someone were to add a little cold water to a well-mixed pool, he would not immediately ruin its good mixture. So, we also say that the environment is well mixed even if it acquires some small change in either direction. And why is it surprising if all grant good mixture

ἄτμητον ὑπάρχειν εἰκός, τὴν μέντοι γ᾽ εἰς χρείαν ἰοῦ-
σαν πλάτος ἔχειν; πολλάκις γὰρ ἡρμόσθαι δοκοῦσαν
ἄριστα λύραν ἕτερος μουσικὸς ἀκριβέστερον ἐφηρ-
μόσατο. πανταχοῦ γὰρ ἡ αἴσθησις ἡμῖν ἐστι κριτήριον
ὡς πρὸς τὰς ἐν τῷ βίῳ χρείας· ὥστε καὶ τὴν εὐκρασίαν δήπου καὶ τὴν δυσκρασίαν αἰσθήσει κρινοῦμεν.

ὡσαύτως δὲ καὶ τὴν τῆς ἐνεργείας βλάβην ἑκάστου τῶν βεβλαμμένων παρὰ τὸ κατὰ φύσιν, ὅταν
εἰς αἰσθητὸν ἥκῃ μέγεθος, ἤδη νόσον ἡμῖν εἶναι νομι-
στέον, οὐδὲν ὡς πρὸς τὰ παρόντα διαφέροντος οὐδ᾽
ἐνταῦθα, πότερον αὐτὰς ταύτας τὰς βεβλαμμένας
ἐνεργείας τὸ νόσημα εἶναι λέγει τις ἢ τὰς διαθέσεις,
ὑφ᾽ ὧν (6.24K) βλάπτονται, ὥσπερ οὐδ᾽ εἰ διαθέσεις
τις ἢ κατασκευὰς ὀνομάζειν ἐθέλοι. διῄρηται γὰρ ἡμῖν
ἑτέρωθι καὶ περὶ τῶνδε καὶ δέδεικται κατὰ τὰς διαθέσεις τε καὶ κατασκευὰς τοῦ σώματος ἥ θ᾽ ὑγεία καὶ
ἡ νόσος, οὐ κατὰ τὰς ἐνεργείας τε καὶ βλάβας αὐτῶν

considerable latitude, given that it is probable that the good harmony in lyres is, I suppose, single and indivisible, yet even this also has latitude in practice? Often, one musician more accurately tunes a harp that already seemed to be perfectly tuned. Our perception is always the means by which we judge the activities[40] of things in real life, so that we also judge "good mixture" and "bad mixture," I suppose, with our perception.

Similarly, whenever the injury of the function of each thing that is injured contrary to nature reaches a perceptible magnitude, then we must consider it a sickness. It makes no difference in the present instance whether one says that the injured functions themselves are the disease, or that the conditions by which **(6.24K)** they are impaired are the disease, just as it makes no difference if someone should wish to call these "conditions" or "constitutions." We discussed these things elsewhere and showed that health

συνιστάμεναι. ἀλλὰ πρός γε τὸ φυλάττειν ὑγείαν ἢ ἰᾶσθαι τὰς νόσους οὐδὲν ἐκ τῆς τούτων ἀκριβείας ὀνινάμεθα. μόνον γὰρ ἀρκεῖ γινώσκειν, ὡς ἡ μὲν κατασκευὴ τοῦ σώματος, αἰτίας λόγον ἔχουσα ὡς πρὸς τὴν ἐνέργειαν, ὁ σκοπὸς τῆς ὑγιεινῆς τε καὶ θεραπευτικῆς ἐστι τέχνης· ταύτην γὰρ ἡμῖν φυλάττειν μὲν ὑπάρχουσαν πρόκειται, δημιουργεῖν δὲ ἀπολλυμένην·

and sickness relate to conditions and constitutions of the body, and not to their functions and injuries. But concerning the preservation of health or the treatment of sickness, we derive no benefit from precision in these matters, since it suffices to recognize only that the constitution of the body, with a causal account in relation to function, is the aim of both the hygienic and the therapeutic arts. Our aim is to maintain health when it is already present and to produce it where it is lost.

On the Differences of Diseases

This text outlines Galen's view of diseases as existing on a spectrum, a perspective undergirded by his theoretical commitments, which locate the origins of disease within the imbalances of humors. He also discusses definitions proposed by rival schools of thought. He divides the body into three substructures: homoiomeric parts, also

(6.836.1K) Πρῶτον μὲν εἰπεῖν χρὴ, τί ποτε νόσημα καλοῦμεν, ἵν' ᾖ δῆλον, ὑπὲρ οὗ σπουδάζει τὸ γράμμα· δεύτερον δ' ἐπὶ τούτῳ, πόσα τὰ σύμπαντά ἐστιν ἁπλᾶ τε καὶ πρῶτα νοσήματα καὶ οἱονεὶ στοιχεῖα τῶν ἄλλων· ἐφεξῆς τε τρίτον, ὁπόσα τὰ ἐκ τούτων συντιθέμενα γίνεται. Ληπτέον δὴ κἀνταῦθα ὁμολογουμένην ἀρχήν, ὡς ἅπαντες ἄνθρωποι, ἐπειδὰν μὲν τὰς

translated as "uniform parts" (that is, ligaments, arteries, veins, bones, nerves, cartilage, membranes, and skin); organs; and the entire body itself. In this section, he outlines his basic definitions of health and disease. As described in the introduction, Galen draws heavily from his philosophical background in these passages, creating fine distinctions among disease categories and developing the foundations of a sophisticated system of diagnosis and disease classification.

DEFINITIONS OF HEALTH AND DISEASE

(6.836.1K) First, we must say what exactly it is that we call a "disease," so that it may be clear what this book endeavors to do. And then next after that, we must say how many simple and primary diseases there are altogether, which are, as it were, the elements of the rest of the diseases. And then third, we must say how many

ἐνεργείας τῶν τοῦ σώματος μορίων εἰς τὰς κατὰ τὸν
βίον πράξεις ὑπηρετούσας ἀμέμπτως ἔχωσιν, ὑγιαίνειν εἰσὶ πεπεισμένοι, βλαβέντες δ' **(6.837K)** ἡντι-
ναοῦν ἐξ αὐτῶν, νοσεῖν ἐκείνῳ τῷ μέρει νομίζουσιν.
εἰ δὲ ταῦθ' οὕτως ἔχει, τὴν ὑγείαν ἐν δυοῖν τούτοιν
ζητητέον, ἢ ἐν ταῖς κατὰ φύσιν ἐνεργείαις, ἢ ἐν ταῖς
κατασκευαῖς τῶν ὀργάνων, ὑφ' ὧν ἐνεργοῦμεν· ὥστε
καὶ ἡ νόσος ἢ ἐνεργείας ἐστὶν, ἢ κατασκευῆς βλάβη.

ἀλλ' ἐπεὶ καὶ κοιμώμενοι, καὶ ἄλλως ἐν σκότῳ καὶ
ἡσυχίᾳ διάγοντες, ἢ κατακείμενοι πολλάκις οὔτε τι
μέρος κινοῦμεν, οὔθ' ὅλως αἰσθανόμεθα τῶν ἔξωθεν
οὐδενός, οὐδὲν μὴν ἧττον ὑγιαίνομεν, κἂν τούτῳ
δῆλον, ὡς οὐ τὸ ἐνεργεῖν ἐστι τὸ ὑγιαίνειν, ἀλλὰ τὸ

diseases there are formed from these simple and primary diseases. We must take as a conventionally accepted starting point here that all people believe they are healthy whenever the functions of their body parts work faultlessly for the activities of life, **(6.837K)** and whenever they are injured in respect of any of these functions, think that they are sick in that part. If this is the case, then health must be sought in those two things, either in functions that are in accordance with nature, or in the constitutions of the organs by which we function. Consequently, sickness too is either an injury in function or an injury in constitution.

But since, too, when we are sleeping or otherwise passing time in darkness and silence or lying down, we often do not move any body part or perceive anything at all that is around us, but no less for that are healthy, it is clear from this that to be healthy is not merely to function,

δύνασθαι. δυνάμεθα δὲ ἐνεργεῖν ἐκ τῆς κατὰ φύσιν κατασκευῆς· ἐν ταύτῃ ἄρα τὸ ὑγιαίνειν ἐστίν. ἕξει δὴ λόγον αἰτίας ἡ κατασκευὴ πρὸς τὴν ἐνέργειαν· ὥστ᾽, εἴτε τὴν κατὰ φύσιν ἁπάντων τῶν μορίων κατασκευὴν ὑγείαν ὀνομάζειν ἐθέλοις, εἴτε τὴν τῶν ἐνεργειῶν αἰτίαν, εἰς ταὐτὸν ἄμφω τὼ λόγω συμβαίνουσιν.

ἀλλ᾽ εἴπερ ἡ ὑγεία τοῦτο, δῆλον ὡς ἡ νόσος τὸ ἐναντίον, ἤτοι κατασκευή τις παρὰ φύσιν, ἢ βλάβης ἐνεργείας αἰτία. δῆλον δὲ ὡς, εἰ καὶ διάθεσιν εἴποις παρὰ (6.838K) φύσιν, ὀνόματί τε χρήσῃ παλαιῷ καὶ δηλώσεις ταὐτό. κατὰ πόσους δὲ τρόπους ἐξιστάμενα τὰ σώματα τοῦ κατὰ φύσιν ἐμποδίζεται περὶ τὰς ἐνεργείας, εἴπερ εὕροιμεν, οὕτως ἂν ἤδη τὸν ἀριθμὸν ἁπάντων τῶν ἁπλῶν νοσημάτων εὑρηκότες εἴημεν.

but rather to be capable of functioning. We are capable of functioning on the basis of the constitution that accords with nature.[41] "Being healthy," then, consists in this. The constitution will in fact have a causal account in relation to the function, so that whether you wish to call health "a constitution of all parts according with nature" or "the cause of functions," both arguments lead to the same conclusion.

But if this is health, it is clear that sickness is its opposite, that is, either some constitution contrary to nature or the cause of an injury in function. And it is also clear that, even if you were to say "condition contrary to **(6.838K)** nature," you will be using an old-fashioned term but will be setting forth the same point. If we were to discover how many ways that bodies, departing from their respective natures, are impaired in their functions, in that way we would

ἀρχὴ δὲ κἀνταῦθα ὁμολογουμένη, σύμμετρον μὲν εἶναι τὸ κατὰ φύσιν οὐκ ἐν ζώῳ μόνον, ἀλλὰ καὶ ἐν φυτῷ καὶ σπέρματι καὶ ὀργάνῳ παντί, τὸ δὲ αὖ παρὰ φύσιν ἄμετρον. εἴη ἂν οὖν ἡ μὲν ὑγεία συμμετρία τις, ἡ δὲ νόσος ἀμετρία. τίνων οὖν ἡ νόσος ἀμετρία, σκεπτέον ἐφεξῆς. ἢ δηλονότι, ὧνπερ ἡ ὑγεία συμμετρία, τούτων ἡ νόσος ἀμετρία; εἰ μὲν οὖν ἐν πόρων συμμετρίᾳ τὸ ὑγιαίνειν ἐστίν, ἐν πόρων ἀμετρίᾳ γενήσεται καὶ τὸ νοσεῖν· εἰ δ᾽ ἐν εὐκρασίᾳ θερμοῦ καὶ ψυχροῦ καὶ ξηροῦ καὶ ὑγροῦ τὸ ὑγιαίνειν ἐστίν, ἐν τῇ τούτων δυσκρασίᾳ καὶ τὸ νοσεῖν ἐξ ἀνάγκης συμβήσεται.

then also have discovered the number of all the simple diseases that exist.

Another conventionally agreed starting point is that what accords with nature is well balanced, not only in an animal but also in a plant, seed, every organ, and, conversely, that what is contrary to nature is imbalanced. So, health therefore would be a certain good balance, and sickness a lack of balance. We must next investigate what things disease is an imbalance of. Or is it clear that, whatever things health is a good balance of, sickness is an imbalance of those same things? So, if being healthy consists in a good balance of pores, then being sick too will consist in an imbalance of the pores,[42] or if being healthy consists in a good mixture of hot, cold, wet, and dry, then it will necessarily follow that sickness consists in a bad mixture of these same things.

NOTES

1. Thomas Kuhn, *Structure of Scientific Revolutions*, rev. and updated ed. (Chicago: University of Chicago Press, 2012).

2. There are some exceptions to this exclusion from modern practice. In his 2020 biography of Galen (*Galen: A Thinking Doctor in Imperial Rome*), Vivian Nutton describes how some of Galen's theoretical principles are still studied in very different contexts, including in Yunani (the Arabic word for "Ionian," that is, Greek) medicine, in certain branches of Tibetan medicine, and even in modern Western contexts that focus on holistic or alternative therapeutic approaches (see Nutton, *Galen: A Thinking Doctor in Imperial Rome*, 1).

3. The complete text is preserved in Arabic. For
   the critical edition and the English translation
   from which this quote has been adapted, see
   Iskandar, *Galeni de optimo medico cognoscendo*; and for discussion of dates of composi-
   tion, see Iskandar, *Galeni de optimo medico
   cognoscendo*, 30–34.

4. Singer, *Galen: Selected Works*, xiv–xxxix.

5. See *Affections and Errors*, 5.41–43K (translation in Singer, *Galen: Psychological Writings*,
   272–74).

6. For an extended description of the philosophers
   and physicians with whom Galen studied,
   see chapter 2 of Susan Mattern's *The Prince of
   Medicine*.

7. The literature around questions of causality in
   Greek philosophical and medical thought is extensive and complex, and I here of necessity present an oversimplification. For an overview of

this topic, see Hankinson, *Cause and Explanation in Ancient Greek Thought*.

8. For more information about these anatomical investigations, see von Staden, *Herophilus*, as well as Nutton, *Ancient Medicine*. Besides dissection of cadavers, these individuals also likely practiced vivisection.

9. Mattern, *Prince of Medicine*, 204.

10. Theriac was a complicated mixture of spices and animal products (including, by Galen's time, viper's flesh) that was initially developed by the kings of Pontus in the second century BCE. It was intended as a prophylactic and antidote for poison, as well as a general therapeutic. Marcus Aurelius took the mixture daily, necessitating its secure and reliable production.

11. Galen's failure to appreciate the closed, integrated nature of the human circulatory system would not be corrected for nearly a millennium

and a half, with the publication of William Harvey's *De Motu Cordis* (*On the Motion of the Heart*) in 1628.

12. For an overview of some of these humoral theories, see Nutton, *Ancient Medicine*, as well as Elizabeth Craik, *The Hippocratic Corpus: Content and Context* (London: Routledge, 2015), especially in both works the sections on the Hippocratic text called *The Nature of Man.*

13. Diogenes, a philosopher active in the fourth century BCE, was notorious for his extreme asceticism: reportedly, he lived in a large wine jar to accustom himself to the harshness of the elements, begged for food, disdained physical possessions, and openly mocked those with money and power (among them, Alexander the Great).

14. The manuscript tradition of this text is extremely problematic, and even the title of the text is interpreted differently in various editions. One way to represent the extended title is

On the Diagnosis and Treatment of the Affections and Errors Peculiar to Each Person's Soul, as Singer has done in *Galen: Psychological Writings.* I use a shortened version of this longer title, *Affections and Errors of the Soul.*

15. "Affections" is a somewhat stilted and technical translation for the Greek πάθος (*pathos*), which could also be translated "suffering," "passion," or even "illness." Galen uses the term in a way that draws on earlier Stoic conceptions of *pathos* as the soul's inappropriate response to external circumstances, while also maintaining the word's connotation of "illness" or "ailment." For further exploration of the philosophical concepts at work here, see Singer, *Galen: Psychological Writings.*

16. "The Pythian oracle" refers to the oracle at the Temple of Apollo in Delphi, a woman who, in an elaborate ritual, would provide often cryptic answers to questions posed by individuals and

governmental delegations alike. In the courtyard of the temple, three short maxims were inscribed on a column, one of which was "Know thyself." I have removed De Boer's parentheticals in this sentence.

17. This phrase is problematic, and Singer has not translated it. I have kept De Boer's text as it is and attempted an interpretation for the first clause. Like Singer, I have omitted (from the Greek text) and not translated <εἰ> καὶ μεῖ[ζ]όν γ' ἐλλιπὲς <τὸ μὴ> ἀποφυγεῖν αὐτά, διότι μικρά.

18. This translation accepts as a conjecture the words κακῶν μεστὴν, as discussed in Singer's *Galen: Psychological Writings*, 243n33, although I have not included these words in the Greek text.

19. The text here is problematic, and I follow Singer's interpretation in *Galen: Psychological Writings*.

20. Thersites is a character in the *Iliad* whose name became, in subsequent Greek literature, a by-word for both physical and moral ugliness. Presented as stupid and obscene, he was described as lame, with a collapsed chest and an oddly shaped head.

21. Among the four humors (black bile, blood, yellow bile, and phlegm), black bile was linked with symptoms of depression (hence our English word melancholy, from the Greek for "black bile").

22. Erasistratus (the same individual renowned for his anatomical investigations) had, according to a widely reported story, diagnosed a case of lovesickness through careful attention to a young man's pulse and physical condition whenever his beloved approached.

23. This phrase is a proverb also seen in Plato's *Symposium* 196c.

24. A moment of Galenic disdain. Galen discusses at multiple points throughout his work the dangers of excessive exercise and his low opinion of those who spend too much time (in his view) training for athletic competitions.

25. Here referring to Homer, *Iliad* 9.503, in which Phoenix describes the futility of prayers, personifying them as lame and blind.

26. I have translated this literally; it is difficult to know what exercise Galen is discussing here.

27. In his treatise *Thrasybulus*, Galen discusses how the trainer is skilled in knowing the technique of the exercises and in ensuring that someone does his exercises appropriately. The physician may possess some elements of this knowledge, but his role is more one of treating problems when they arise, than one of maintaining a patient's fitness. In his introduction to the translation for *Thrasybulus*, translator Ian Johnston (who is also a surgeon) likens the dis-

tinction, in our own terms, to that between a physical therapist and a physician. Johnston, *Galen: Hygiene*, vol. 2, *Books 5–6: Thrasybulus, On Exercise with a Small Ball*. The distinction between the cook and the physician is much older and may be found, for example, in Plato's *Gorgias*.

28. It can be challenging to find precisely analogous terms for some of these exercises, so I have been descriptive when rendering names of the exercises into English. See note 17 in Johnston's translation (*Galen: Hygiene*, vol. 2, *Books 1–4*), as well as Christesen and Kyle, *Companion to Sport and Spectacle in Greek and Roman Antiquity*.

29. For more extensive discussion, see Singer and van der Eijk, *Galen: Works on Human Nature*, 5–10.

30. Here, Galen uses hypothetical names, like we might use "Tom, Dick, and Harry."

31. A genus is more inclusive than a species. Man to man is comparison within the same species, and man to bee/ant is comparison within the same genus, as all are living creatures. This type of thinking is Aristotelian in origin. Galen clarifies these classifications further below, when he describes how plants are of a higher (more inclusive) genus than one that includes only animals. His use of the terms *genus* and *species* is somewhat similar to, but not the same as, our use of them today.

32. This refers to the Hippocratic text *On Nutriment*, section 19.

33. "Units" here is a generic term used in the context of a thought experiment; there was no formal unit system for ranking degrees of mixture.

34. I have translated συμμετρία, from which we have the word "symmetry," as "good balance" to capture its sense not just of proportionality, but of good and appropriate proportionality.

35. The categorical descriptor "white" is a standard predicate in Greek philosophical works on categories and is not to be understood in racial terms.

36. Galen is inserting differences in terminology that are used by different medical sects.

37. This is Galen's rebuttal to those who argue that the body is perpetually affected by disease.

38. Although it may seem that Galen is gesturing toward what we might call germ theory, ideas of contagion in antiquity were very different from our own. For further discussion of this topic, see Vivian Nutton, "The Seeds of Disease: An Explanation of Contagion and Infection from the Greeks to the Renaissance," *Medical History* 27 (1983): 1–24.

39. These are all Greek mythological figures legendary for the abilities with which they are paired here.

40. I have translated χρεία variably ("use," "practice," or "activity"), depending on the context.

41. Here, Galen is describing health as an individual's particular constitution that is at its baseline, natural condition. I follow Johnston, *Galen: On Diseases and Symptoms*, here in rendering ἐκ τῆς κατὰ φύσιν κατασκευῆς as "constitution that accords with nature."

42. Galen's mention of "pores" is a reference to another school of medical thought and practice, described further in Nutton, *Ancient Medicine*, 171.

SOURCE TEXTS

Avoiding Distress

Source of the text: Boudon-Millot, Véronique, Jacques Jouanna, and Antoine Pietrobelli. *Galien*. Vol. 4, *Ne pas se chagriner*. Collection Budé. Paris: Les Belles Lettres, 2010.

Other textual editions: Garofalo, Ivan, Anna Maria Urso, Klaus-Dietrich Fischer, Vito Lorusso, Alessandro Lami, and Nicoletta Palmieri. "Congetture e emendamenti inediti," *Galenos* 4 (2010): 267–78.

Garofalo, Ivan, and Alessandro Lami. *Galeno: L'anima e il dolore*. Milan: BUR classici greci e latini, 2012.

Other English translations: Vivian Nutton's notes and translation in Singer, Peter, ed. *Galen: Psychological Writings*. Cambridge: Cambridge University Press, 2013.

Affections and Errors of the Soul

Source of the text: CMG V 4,1,1. De Boer, Wilko. *Galeni De propriorum animi cuiuslibet affectuum dignotione et curatione; De animi cuiuslibet peccatorum dignotione et curatione; De atra bile*. Leipzig: Berlin-Brandenburg Academy of Sciences, 1937. I have made a few changes in punctuation.

Kühn reference: 5.1–103; sections included in this translation are 5.2.14–5.15.5.

Numbering: Numbers ending with "D" are according to De Boer's text, by page and line number, separated with a period; higher numbers (written with a "K") correspond to Kühn. Some paragraph designations and some small changes to punctuation are my own.

Other English translations: Singer, Peter. *Galen: Psychological Writings*, Cambridge: Cambridge University Press, 2013.

Prognosis, for Epigenes

Source of the text: CMG V 8,1. Nutton, Vivian. *Galeni De Praecognitione*. Berlin: Akademie Verlag, 1979.

Kühn reference: 14.599–673; translated section is 14.631.5–14.633.13.

Numbering: Numbers written with a "K" correspond to Kühn, as also reproduced in Nutton's volume. Some paragraph designations and some small changes to punctuation are my own.

Other English translations: Nutton's edition, above, under "Source of the text," includes an English translation.

On Exercise with a Small Ball

Source of the text: Wenkebach, Ernst. *Sudhoff's Archiv für Geschichte der Medizin und der Naturwissenschaften* 31, no. 4/5 (September 1938): 254–97.

Kühn reference: 5.899–910; the entire passage is translated.

Numbering: Single-digit numbers are those according to Wenkebach's text; the higher numbers (written with a "K") correspond to Kühn. The paragraph designations and some small changes to punctuation are my own.

Other English translations: Singer, Peter. *Galen: Selected Works*. Oxford: Oxford University Press, 1997.

Johnston, Ian. *Galen: Hygiene*, Vol. 2, Books 5–6. *Thrasybulus. On Exercise with a Small Ball*. Loeb Classical Library. Cambridge, MA: Harvard University Press, 2018.

On Hygiene

Source of the text: Koch, Konrad. CMG V 4.2. *Galeni de sanitate tuenda*. Leipzig: Teubner, 1923.

Kühn reference: 6.1–6.452 for the entire text; translated section is 6.139.9–6.147.8.

Numbering: Numbers written with a "K" correspond to Kühn, a notation that Koch also uses. Some paragraph designations and some small changes to punctuation are my own.

Other English translations: Johnston, Ian.
Galen: Hygiene, Vol. 1, Books 1–4. Loeb Classical
Library. Cambridge, MA: Harvard University
Press, 2018.

Mixtures 1.5 and 2.4

Source of the text: Helmreich, Georg. *Galenus:
De Temperamentis*. Leipzig: Teubner, 1904.
Kühn reference: 1.509–694 for the entire text; ex-
cerpts from 1.544.16–1.548.5 and 1.609.1–1.610.4.
Numbering: Numbers written with a "K" corre-
spond to Kühn. The paragraph designations and
some small changes to punctuation are my own.
Other translations: Singer, Peter. *Galen: Selected
Works*. Oxford: Oxford University Press, 1997.

On the Properties of Foods

Source of the text: Wilkins, John. *Galien*. Vol. 5,
Sur les facultés des aliments. Collection Budé. Paris:
Les Belles Lettres, 2013.

Kühn reference: 6.453–748 for entire text; translated sections are 6.453.2–6.454.3; 6.464.15–6.465.13; 6.467.14–6.470.4.

Numbering: Numbers written with a "K" correspond to Kühn. Some paragraph designations and some small changes to punctuation are my own.

Other English translations: Grant, Mark. *Galen on Food and Diet*. London: Routledge, 2000.

On Hygiene

Source of the text: Koch, Konrad. CMG V 4.2. *Galeni de sanitate tuenda*. Leipzig: Teubner, 1923.

Kühn reference: 6.1–452 for the entire text; translated section is 6.13.8–6.24.10.

Numbering: Numbers written with a "K" correspond to Kühn. The paragraph designations and some small changes to punctuation are my own.

Other English translations: Johnston, Ian. *Galen: Hygiene*, Vol. 1, Books 1–4. Loeb Classical Library. Cambridge, MA: Harvard University Press, 2018.

On the Differences of Diseases

Source of the text: Kühn 6.836–6.880; translated section is 6.836.1–6.839.1.

Other translations: Johnston, Ian. *Galen: On Diseases and Symptoms*. Cambridge: Cambridge University Press, 2006.

FURTHER READING

As described in the introduction, the Galenic corpus is vast, and so is the volume of secondary literature devoted to understanding this fascinating physician, his ideas, and the reception of Galenism across time and space. Below are several books that may serve as starting points for further exploration, as well as references to the critical editions from which the Greek text in this volume was sourced. Additional references are given in the notes.

General Overviews of Galen and His World

Gill, Christopher, Tim Whitmarsh, and John Wilkins. *Galen and the World of Knowledge*. Cambridge: Cambridge University Press, 2009.

Hankinson, Robert. *The Cambridge Companion to Galen*. Cambridge: Cambridge University Press, 2008.

Mattern, Susan. *Galen and the Rhetoric of Healing*. Baltimore: Johns Hopkins University Press, 2008.

———. *The Prince of Medicine: Galen in the Roman Empire*. Oxford: Oxford University Press, 2013.

Nutton, Vivian. *Ancient Medicine*. 2nd ed. London: Routledge, 2013.

———. *Galen: A Thinking Doctor in Imperial Rome*. London: Taylor and Francis, 2020.

Selected Texts on Greco-Roman Medicine and Philosophy

Hankinson, Robert, *Cause and Explanation in Ancient Greek Thought*. Oxford: Oxford University Press, 2001.

Jouanna, Jacques. *Hippocrates*. Translated into English by M. B. DeBevoise. Baltimore: Johns Hopkins University Press, 1999.

FURTHER READING

von Staden, Heinrich. *Herophilus: The Art of Medicine in Early Alexandria*. Cambridge: Cambridge University Press, 1989.

Sport and Exercise in Greco-Roman Antiquity

Christesen, Paul, and Donald Kyle. *A Companion to Sport and Spectacle in Greek and Roman Antiquity*. Chichester: Wiley Blackwell, 2014.

Textual Editions

The Corpus Medicorum Graecorum (CMG), published by the Berlin-Brandenburg Academy of Sciences, provides comprehensive and up-to-date editions and translations (into German, English, French, and Italian) of the texts of Greco-Roman medical authors, including Galen (https://cmg.bbaw .de/en/homepage). Source languages are not limited to Greek and Latin but also include Arabic, Hebrew, Latin, and Syriac. These volumes are cited with reference to their CMG volume number. The

French press Les Belle Lettres has also published a number of critical editions of texts of Galen in its Collection Budé series.

Boudon-Millot, Véronique, Jacques Jouanna, and Antoine Pietrobelli. *Galien*. Vol. 4, *Ne pas se chagriner*. Collection Budé. Paris: Les Belles Lettres, 2010.

De Boer, Wilko. *Galeni De propriorum animi cuius-libet affectuum dignotione et curatione; De animi cuiuslibet peccatorum dignotione et curatione; De atra bile*. Leipzig: Berlin-Brandenburg Academy of Sciences, 1937.

Garofalo, Ivan, and Alessandro Lami. *Galeno: L'anima e il dolore*. Milan: BUR classici greci e latini, 2012.

Helmreich, Georg. *Galeni De temperamentis libri III*. Leipzig: Teubner, 1904.

Iskandar, Albert. CMG Suppl. Or. IV, *Galeni de optimo medico cognoscendo*. Berlin: Akademie Verlag, 1988.

Koch, Konrad. CMG V 4,2, *Galeni De sanitate tuenda libri VI*. Leipzig: Teubner, 1923.

Kühn, Carl Gottlob. *Claudii Galeni opera omnia*. 22 vols. Leipzig: Knobloch, 1821–33; reprinted Hildesheim: Georg Olms Verlag, 1964–65.

Nutton, Vivian. CMG V 8,1, *Galeni De Praecognitione*. Berlin: Akademie Verlag, 1979.

Wenkebach, Ernst. "Galenos von Pergamon: Allgemeine Ertüchtigung durch Ballspiel; Eine sporthygienische Schrift aus dem zweiten Jahrhundert n. Chr." *Sudhoff's Archiv für Geschichte der Medizin und der Naturwissenschaften* 31, no. 4/5 (1938): 254–97. Available on the CMG website.

Wilkins, John. *Galien*. Vol. 5, *Sur les facultés des aliments*. Collection Budé. Paris: Belles Lettres, 2013.

English Translations

This list includes additional English translations of the full texts associated with the excerpts I have translated and provided in this book. Note that these also provide substantial and informative introductory overviews to the texts. Singer's Cambridge

University Press editions also provide helpful glossaries showing original Greek words, transliterated Greek words, and the corresponding English translation.

Grant, Mark. *Galen on Food and Diet*. London: Routledge, 2000.

Johnston, Ian. *Galen: On Diseases and Symptoms*. Cambridge: Cambridge University Press, 2006.

———. *Galen: Hygiene*, Vol. 1, Books 1–4. Loeb Classical Library. Cambridge, MA: Harvard University Press, 2018.

———. *Galen: Hygiene*, Vol. 2, Books 5–6. *Thrasybulus. On Exercise with a Small Ball*. Loeb Classical Library. Cambridge, MA: Harvard University Press, 2018.

Powell, Owen, and John Wilkins. *Galen: On the Properties of Foodstuffs*. Cambridge: Cambridge University Press, 2003.

Singer, Peter. *Galen: Selected Works*. Oxford: Oxford University Press, 1997.

———. *Galen: Psychological Writings*. Cambridge: Cambridge University Press, 2013.

Singer, Peter, and Philip van der Eijk. *Galen: Works on Human Nature*. Cambridge: Cambridge University Press, 2018.